Internationally Respected
Instructors Offer Accolades for

Welcome To Karate

This is information that beginners need. It is clear and easy to read and understand. I would recommend this book to new students.

— James Field, 8th Dan
Member, ISKF Shihankai
Vice-Chairman, ISKF Technical Committee
Chief Instructor, ISKF Southwest Region USA

Since getting my hands on Bruce Costa's Welcome To Karate, *I have dipped into it on many occasions. It is full of little gems, small bits of advice, and tips to help a karate-ka get the most from their training. Designed and written with the beginner in mind, it still offers insights for practitioners of all levels.*

Bruce cleverly recognises that "we keep our karate in a handy, portable, carry-all container," we are able to practise anywhere, anytime. I would go one step further and say that within this little, handy, portable book is a wealth of knowledge that will help the self-practicing karateka get even more from their endeavours.

— Scott Langley, 6th Dan
Founder, HDKI
Chief Instructor, Hombu Dojo Karate, Ireland
Author of *Karate Stupid* and *Karate Clever*

Very thoughtful presentation and great information. I love your enthusiasm and spirit.

— Rick Hotton, 5th Dan
Founder, Sunday Morning Keiko
Chief Instructor, West Wind Dojo
Creator of *Holy Molé*

Welcome To Karate *is a valuable addition to the current karate literature. Karate instructor Bruce Costa, drawing on his many years of karate teaching experience, has put together a manual that will assist beginners in understanding the traditions and practices of Shotokan karate. Many of these traditions are overlooked in other karate manuals and it is refreshing to see that Mr. Costa has emphasized them in order to preserve the traditions*

of this supreme martial art. Beginners entering the dojo would be well advised to refer to this book for a complete understanding of the art that they are about to undertake. Further, his discussion of basic techniques makes them comprehensible to new students. This is, I feel, a very important part of this book. It should be mandatory reading for all new students. I strongly recommend it to students and instructors alike.

— Robin Reilly, 8th Dan
Member, ISKF Shihankai
Chairman, ECSKA Technical Committee
Chief Instructor, Kobukan Karate Club
Author of 11 books, including *Complete Shotokan Karate* and *Karate for Kids*

One of the fascinating things about karate is that no matter how long we train, there is always something to be learned. Thank you for the time and energy you devoted to providing us a fresh, new approach.

— Najib Amin, 8th Dan
Member, ISKF Technical Committee
Chief Instructor, Shotokan Karate Club of Maryland

...I read your book cover to cover on the plane ride home. It is very well done and I enjoyed it very much. I think you did a thorough job of covering all aspects of training and etiquette that are needed to train in a dojo. I was happy to see the principles of respect and diligence emphasized in the training and the explanations. I will review it again and share it with a couple of my senior students . . . Good work . . .

— Cathy Cline, 8th Dan
Member, ISKF Technical Committee
Chief Instructor, Western Washington Shotokan Karate Club
Highest-Ranked Woman in the World

I congratulate you on a great book, very well written and full of great knowledge that not only 9th kyus need to know, but the rest of us karateka.

— Mark Willis, 8th Dan
Deputy Chief Instructor, Traditional Shotokan KarateDo Federation
ISKF New Zealand

Sensei Costa has cleverly filled the gap for concise, thoughtful, and meaningful reading material for those embarking upon their journey into traditional karate. His work introduces the concepts, principles, and subtle nuances of karate as it is practiced in dojos across the globe. It is a gem of a book that I am thrilled to recommend to anyone interested in practicing karate. Well done indeed!

— David Jones, 8th Dan
Member, ISKF Technical Committee
Regional Director, ISKF Canada
Chief Instructor, ISKF Alberta

[Welcome To Karate] *is a good book, very high quality.*

— Oded Friedman, 8th Dan
Regional Director and Technical Committee CEO
ISKF Israel

It is clear that Mr. Costa has spent countless hours-developing this concise and well-written piece on traditional karate-do. It was a pleasure to read and in fact helped me re-evaluate some very important points. I would highly recommend adding this to your library on martial arts training.

— Bob Hoffman, 8th Dan
Chairman, East Coast Region ISKF Technical Committee
Chief Instructor, Chester County Shotokan Karate Club

[Welcome To Karate] *is a great support for teaching. I even gave it to my students who teach in different dojos to help them. I thank you!*

— Fady Antakly, 7th Dan
Regional Director, ISKF Lebanon

I congratulate Bruce on this well thought-out, very useful book…it provides beginners with valuable information on studying the martial art of karate-do. I highly recommend this book.

— Larry Loreth, 8th Dan
Member, ISKF Technical Committee
President, ISKF Canada
Chief Instructor, ISKF Manitoba

Bruce Costa has written an excellent manual for the beginning karate student. Welcome To Karate *not only covers all the technical material a beginning student needs to know, but it also covers the etiquette and social aspects of beginning karate lessons. I particularly like the helpful self-training tips sprinkled throughout the text. Any beginning student can use this manual to ease what can be an awkward and intimidating first step into the dojo. I would have like to have such a text available when I started karate and would recommend this book to my beginning karate students without reservation.*

— Paul Willoughby, 5th Dan
Chief Instructor, Southern Maryland Shotokan Karate

Welcome To Karate *has helped our son realize the importance of every aspect of his karate, to understand what it means to be mindful of his actions, more present in the moment, and respectful of others.*

— Brenda Staehle
mother of Brandon, Purple Belt

Welcome To
KARATE

Unlocking the Wisdom of
the Beginner's Mind

BRUCE COSTA

YMAA Publication Center
Wolfeboro, NH USA

YMAA Publication Center, Inc.
PO Box 480
Wolfeboro, NH 03894
800 669-8892 • www.ymaa.com • info@ymaa.com

ISBN: 9781594398414 (print) • ISBN: 9781594398421 (ebook)
This book set in Optima, Alexa, and Zapfino.
Edited by Doran Hunter.
Cover adaptation by Axie Breen based upon Bruce Costa's original design.
Photography and photo editing by Aaron Mitchell Photography.
Original Heian Shodan diagram ©Albrecht Pflüger, used with permission. Adapted for an
English-speaking audience by Bruce Costa.
Dachi, Tai Sabaki, and Embusen diagrams by Bruce Costa.
Illustrations provided by the author unless otherwise noted.

20210901

Publisher's Cataloging in Publication

Names:	Costa, Bruce Guido, 1961- author. ∣ Okazaki, Teruyuki, 1931-2020 writer of foreword.
Title:	Welcome to karate : unlocking the wisdom of the beginner's mind / Bruce Costa ; foreword by Teruyuki Okazaki.
Other titles:	Unlocking the wisdom of the beginner's mind.
Description:	Wolfeboro, NH USA : YMAA Publication Center, [2021] ∣ Series: Welcome to karate.
Identifiers:	ISBN: 97815943988414 (print) ∣ 9781594398421 (ebook) ∣ LCCN: 2021941401
Subjects:	LCSH: Karate--Handbooks, manuals, etc. ∣ Karate--Training. ∣ Martial arts--Training. ∣ Stretching exercises. ∣ Muscle strength. ∣ Qi (Chinese philosophy) ∣ BISAC: HEALTH & FITNESS / Exercise / Stretching. ∣ SPORTS & RECREATION / Martial Arts / General.
Classification:	LCC: GV1114.3 .C67 2021 ∣ DDC: 796.815/3--dc23

Printed in Canada.

With good reason, I dedicate this book to my three grown children.

Among we who've founded martial arts schools, how many were young parents at the time? The benefit of that stoic lifestyle is the birthright of our daughters and sons…but they didn't ask. Therefore, for having undertaken their father's requirements with aplomb, I offer this book to Granite Forest Dojo's excellent first three students:
Alexandria, Zachariah, and Samantha Costa.

They are most precious to me.

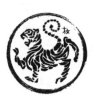

CONTENTS

FOREWORD BY TERUYUKI OKAZAKI

Founder, International Shotokan Karate Federation

It is with pleasure that I submit the foreword to this handbook by Mr. Bruce Costa. It is always heartwarming for me when a student of mine not only continues to train but also makes the decision to share their experience and training with others. Bruce first began his Shotokan karate training with me as a student at Temple University. Many university students, once they finish their academic commitment, discontinue their karate training. However, it is fortunate for the many students Bruce has guided in the karate community that he remained true to this martial art.

This manual is a helpful tool for the beginner student. It explains the proper *dojo* etiquette as well as the basic *kihon*, *kata*, and *kumite*. It is always beneficial to guide the beginner student to what they can expect on a journey they will hopefully continue for their entire lives. What is most important for them to remember is that we never stop learning.

Studying martial arts is a life-long endeavor. You are never finished, and there is no graduation. This is because the hardest technique you will ever have to study diligently is to do your best to strive to attain your main goal, which is perfection of character. This can only be achieved if you do your best to live by the *Dojo Kun* and the *niju kun*. These guidelines will help you to be a good martial artist and a good human being. When you open your mind to accept these precepts, you will then begin to learn how to be a true martial artist. In the dojo, you are learning the tools to protect yourself and your family. But you are also learning the tools to be a good human being. You must train hard and keep your Dojo Kun not only in the dojo but also in your everyday life. When you treat others with respect and courtesy, they will respond to you in the same manner.

Respect and courtesy are contagious. When we treat each other this way, we will be making a contribution to making the world a better place. This is our ultimate goal.

Author's note: Throughout his adult life and throughout the world, Grand Master Teruyuki Okazaki (岡崎 照幸, June 22, 1931 —April 21, 2020, student of Gichin Funakoshi and Masatoshi Nakayama) was respected not only for his position, but for his legendary skill in kara-te. During the four decades I benefitted from his mentorship, I came to understand how his generous grace and good humor were equally deserving of such high regard. For all these reasons and more, his willingness to compose a foreword for this small book has been my profound honor.

Early in my practice, "Sensei" (as we all singularly called him in those days; every other teacher was "Mr." or "Ms.") provided my first exposure to the concept he called soshin ni kaeru, *wherein we were to conceptually return to a time before having learned, in order to have the most receptive possible attitude. To this day, such open-mindedness enables me to attend classes I'm supposedly overqualified for and pick up new information. It works every time. I have used this skill in countless areas of my life. It is the reason for the subtitle of this book.*

Thank you, Sensei.

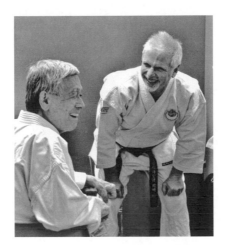

The ultimate aim of the art of karate lies not in victory or defeat but in the perfection of the character of its participants.

Master Gichin Funakoshi

GRATITUDE

I am fortunate beyond words, but they will have to do.

I begin with the team I'm so happy to have joined, especially YMAA publisher David Ripianzi, editor Doran Hunter, typesetter Tim Comrie, designer Axie Breen, and publicist Gene Ching. In addition to their decades-honed professionalism, they've brought me hours of happy martial arts philosophizing. I await many more as we bring you the *Welcome To Karate* book series.

Having had the pleasure of training in fine martial arts schools throughout multiple countries, I am qualified to tell you that my best experiences have occurred at the one I regularly teach in. This has little to do with me and everything to do with the students and friends I am blessed with there.

Of them, the cream has truly risen to the top. I could not have hand-selected a finer group of seniors to lead the school by example. Of that group, the following have criticized their sensei (no easy task for a dedicated karateka, and they all are) in an effort to make this a better book.

Terence Farrell	James Viscusi, Jr
Sandra Viscusi	Barbara Conroy
Stacy Zeller	Samantha Zeller
George McKnight	Brenda Staehle

I'm also appreciative of my students who brought the concepts described in this book to life. In order of appearance, they are Julia Quinn, Akinbode Akinkunmi, Aavni Sitapara, Daniel Elliott, Lincoln Elliott, Aleia Castro, Nathan Wampole, Jibril Heckler, Mikail Heckler, Joseph Quinn, Elijah Elliott, Ethan Kim, Barbara Conroy, Luca Lombardo, Benjamin Jordan, Thomas Heckler, Ava Komasz, Samantha Costa, and Tilly Strunk. I am especially grateful to photomaster Aaron Castro for his remarkable expertise, superb studio, endless good humor, and peanut butter and jelly sandwiches.

HOW TO USE THIS BOOK

This book is meant to do a couple of things. Those things are specific and limited.

First, I hope it will make the very concept of practicing karate a bit less intimidating. You may be watching senior members of your school perform miracles with seeming ease and wondering how you'll ever reach that point. Try to understand: every one of them were once where you are now.

Almost daily in class, at the end of a drill, a blush-faced, winded new student exudes frustration. I offer some tips, perhaps a simple foot placement or shifting of weight, that will make the drill less strenuous and its lessons easier to grasp. At that moment I'll sometimes perceive *more* frustration, as if this person should have been born with such knowledge and, therefore, be performing at black-belt level immediately. When I sense this, in a voice loud enough for the class to hear, I mock gently, "Don't worry! *No* one else in this class has *ever* made the mistakes *you're* making!" It is always a pleasure to watch faces twist and smirk, with an affirming yet somewhat sheepish reply of "osu!" shouted most confidently by those holding the highest rank. It is one of the many advantages of becoming a Black Belt: by then, the karate student has elevated the practice of embarrassing himself to a high art.

Know that yours is a well-tread path. Forgive yourself your mistakes. Indeed, try so hard as to make many of them. Then release your critique of yourself to those who've done this for a while. Your dojo is an institution of learning, perhaps unlike any other you have attended in Western society. Remain quiet, and do

Watch for blocks of text like this one. They provide practical advice for ways to bring your training with you.

Self-Training

Fortunately, we keep our karate in a handy, portable, carry-all container. It requires no particular equipment or facility. At all times, it's ready-to-go.

From this standpoint, karate is among the easiest-to-practice skills you'll ever try to develop. You can fit it into small spaces in your life, like while you're shopping. I like sneaking in a newly learned drill while shopping in the produce section of the supermarket: plenty of space in the wider aisles. Aghast shoppers are a bonus.

all that is asked of you. When you return home, let this book (and its pronunciation guide!) provide you with the comfort of a few more insights regarding your experiences in karate class.

This book's second, more important purpose is to help you bring your karate outside of the dojo. This planet needs to be populated with people possessing insights such as those you'll gain there.

Imagine that you took guitar lessons and, after the first half-hour lesson, your teacher said, "Okay, leave your guitar here. Don't do anything on your own. We'll resume your practice when I see you next time." This is an approach that would guarantee failure, yet it is the one used by most new karate students. Your guitar teacher would serve you better by expecting you to practice every day, even if just for a few minutes. The same is true of your karate teacher. All good karate students self-train. Great karate students self-train daily. There are boxes throughout this book like the one at the top of this page. They will offer materials for your self-training to supplement those received in class.

This book is not to be used without the supervision and guidance of a properly ranked Shotokan karate instructor. It is a supplement to such instruction, not a replacement for it. Indeed, there are countless nuances and details involved in the personal development realized through karate. No one book, or series or collection of books, can replace a good sensei. Active counsel must be provided by someone who has received such guidance through his or her own process of development. At best, this book will provide you with good discussion material, but you need a mentor for such discussions. Your first task, then, if you haven't done so already, is to find a good karate teacher and show him or her respect and gratitude.

A STYLE GUIDE

There are challenges that come with mixing technical Japanese terminology in an English text written for Western audiences. Choices need to be made. I've become convinced that the best possible outcome must result in numerous awkward phraseologies. Nevertheless, we made the best choices we could, two of which I'll explain here.

The plural of Japanese words normally remains unchanged from the singular. If I wanted to explain a trip to the dojo to perform a kata, I would describe the experience with the same words as if I went to several dojo and performed many kata. During a relaxed reading of this text, however, I found myself tripping with every occurrence like a track runner mistiming a hurdle. We will, therefore and not at all smoothly, be going to dojos to perform katas.

The second of these choices involves the use of Japanese. It is not a spoken or written language familiar to most people living in the West, to whom this book series is primarily directed. (Despite whatever awareness of technical terms I possess, it remains a language unfamiliar to me as well, as it does most longtime American practitioners of Japanese martial arts.) In most written works, a word from a language foreign to the reader is italicized. Were we to do that here, however, you'd find yourself in a flurry of tilted senseis, dojos, and other terms familiar even to the disinterested. Therefore, the first appearance of a given Japanese word will be italicized, but it will be presented in normal type thereafter.

BANZAI!

Congratulations!

If you've never set foot in a *dojo* (a facility for learning Asian arts, literally "Place of The Way"), you may think that opening this book is your first step into the world of karate. If you thought that, you'd be wrong about your karate, perhaps for the first time. Don't worry, you're just at the beginning of your journey. You will be wrong about your karate many, many more times.

Your first karate experience occurred when you first thought about becoming involved with karate. You no doubt fantasized what that involvement would be like, what it would feel like. Such processing was very "Zen" of you. And you were, once again, wrong. Nevertheless, you already have experience with karate, and so, congratulations are in order!

I congratulate you because the moment you stepped onto this path, you elevated yourself beyond the self that you were. There are ramifications. For example, you've taken the first step into the misunderstanding of many of your peers. This can cause indifference in your relationships, even conflict. But it can also bring opportunity and renewal to them. It is for this reason I've chosen *Banzai!* from among the many ways to express congratulations in the extraordinarily expressive language of Japanese: I wish you a long life in this wondrous adventure.

And what an adventure you've chosen! With a voracious appetite for learning, I've sought many new experiences. But I know of none that lets me experience the journey itself in quite the way, and quite so much, as karate training does. More than anything I know of, it proves that the destination is not the thing. In my own training, any time I've gotten myself to think I know what I'm doing, I can depend on finding out I was wrong about it in short order. As I tell my students, once you're signed up and are paying tuition, I only need you to do two things:

1) Show up.

2) Try hard.

Without ever having met you, I can guarantee that if you do those two things, you will measurably—and not at all contrarily—grow in both confidence and humility. One thing doesn't take long to discover: there are so very many facets to this experience that it is, indeed, worthy of a lifetime of study.

That's quite a bit to get your brain around. I will like it very much if, every ten years of your training or so, you come back and reread this page to see if you agree. For now, simply know there is a path before you that leads up a very tall mountain.[1]

Good job showing up.

Now try hard.

Bruce Costa
Bucks County, Pennsylvania

---

1 See the story, "Homage: The Mountain," on page 119.

Chapter 1

What Is Karate?

...since karate training has stressed humility and overcoming oneself as fundamental principles from ancient times, even though one may not be aware of the development, it contributes substantially to the polishing of character.

Master Gichin Funakoshi
from Rentan Goshin Karate Jutsu, 1925

Karate is open mindedness.
Karate is humility.
Karate is learning.
Karate is sweat, endurance, excellence.

Yes, karate is a martial art. Those of us who practice *karate-do* think it is the best of them, distilled by great masters from millennia of personal development to the efficiently focused power that is available to us today. We are invited to train hard; I've never seen a martial art practiced with more intensity than ours. We hone basic techniques with tens of thousands of repetitions. We then strive to bring that level of quality to actual encounters with challenging opponents. Finally, these concepts of focus and intensity must be present when we practice the predetermined sequences of techniques called *kata*, wherein we simulate combat against many antagonists. Through developing technique, conditioning, and clarity of mind, we continually reach new heights we'd never imagined were even possible. This experience is as available to newcomers as it is to senior students, which is one reason the only people impressed with a newly appointed Black Belt are those who are not yet Black Belts themselves. Karate is the practice of beginning, the bringing forth of the truth: we are all beginners.

Happily, there are also things karate is not. It is not arrogant. It is not bigoted. Karate is not stubborn or aggrandizing or violent. Those who bring these qualities into the dojo are not practicing karate while they're there. There is no place in karate for these things.

Karate is good exercise, positive discipline, and productive camaraderie. Most of all, karate is the search for perfection of character.

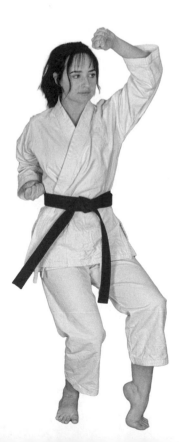

Chapter 2

Empty Your Mind

DOJO ETIQUETTE
Welcome to Japan

To those of us living in the West, used to hugs and handshakes, Eastern etiquette may feel a little … unusual. It seems at times appropriate that our Asian brethren are placed in geographic opposition to us: a Westerner would need to go off-planet to find a culture more dissimilar to his own.

Our use of this etiquette is advantageous because such unfamiliarity offers us a remarkable opportunity. We all start in the same awkward place—entering what may be the largest empty room in our daily lives, bare footed, sporting funny white pajamas, and probably having a look of anxious discomfort. It might be downright embarrassing. I hope you can find reassurance in the understanding that every single person in the *dojo*—from the *sensei* to the most senior *senpai* to the fellow in line next to you wearing the white belt who joined just a few days before you did —*all* of them started with the same unfamiliar feeling. You are invited to do as we did, to see all of this as an invitation to adopt new ways of expressing your humility and to open yourself to a learning method that will let you become your absolute best.

Our humility is found immediately upon entering the karate facility. Traditionally, in Japan and the islands that surround it, one removes one's shoes before entering a home. Here in the West, one can typically enter a facility and locate the appropriate place to remove and store shoes. When I visit a dojo I've never been to before, I take off my shoes before entering. It's just good manners to do so and will save you potential embarrassment if the shoe-removal zone isn't obvious.

After removing shoes and storing any extraneous items, you may need to take care of some administrative business. There may be a sign-in sheet or attendance booklet. Some schools have a computer-entry system, enabling you to record your presence with a keyboard or a card scanner. Our school has a simple index card file box, from which students pull their cards before class. Whatever the method, don't miss this important step. At exam time, you'll want all your attended classes recognized when Sensei is determining your qualifications for promotion.

Your next step will be to "bow onto" the dojo floor. You will learn this very important part of Eastern etiquette in a moment. There are a few details of your participation to be mentioned first, however.

COMPORTMENT

Traditional *Shotokan karateka* (karate practitioners) wear pure white uniforms. This can be puzzling to parents of karate kids who have long considered white a color to be excluded from their child's wardrobe. But your uniform is important in that it signifies the purity of our art. There is no pretension in the dojo; no one practitioner is better dressed than any other. There is only what we bring to the training floor. As is the case everywhere in life (though we sometimes behave as if it isn't so), we are fully responsible for the way we present ourselves. Once we learn these few concepts, the dojo becomes a place for us to comfortably and courteously practice that presentation alongside our peers. We all have the same, clear system of etiquette.

❖ Your *gi* (uniform) should be neat, clean, and odor free. You'll be working closely and intensely with your friends in class; you want them to consider you a friend *after* class as well! Heavier, twelve- to fifteen-ounce cotton uniforms, while preferred for training, are prone to wrinkling. They can be pressed if so desired. To avoid ironing, develop the skill of pulling your gi out of the dryer before the heavy wrinkles set in.

❖ All **jewelry** should be removed, not only because not all of us can afford jewelry but, more importantly, because of safety, primarily your own. Nothing should be worn around your wrist, even a hair band. If removing and replacing a piercing is infeasible, covering and securing the piercing with athletic tape is permissible.

❖ **Fingernails and toenails** *must* be kept short. In the heat of class, when you've been exercising heavily, your skin will be moist, soft, and easily cut. Causing a laceration to a partner with an unkept nail is not only unhygienic, it's just plain inconsiderate. A nick by your nail would require your partner to bow out of class, clean his wound, and bandage it before waiting to be allowed back in, after he went through who-knows-what in his personal life to be present for class. As his partner, you would feel badly costing him any of his training experience because you injured him through discourtesy. At a minimum, groom your nails weekly.

❖ **Hair** should be clean and restricted. Longer hair must be tied up or somehow contained. I've seen flailing hair cause a slight eye wound more than once. More often still, I've seen it occlude vision, resulting in loss of awareness and potential injury. I consider it enough of a safety issue to keep a basket of clips, ties, and bobby pins at the edge of our training floor for this purpose. Courteously restrain your hair and make it a non-issue for yourself and others before class begins.

The result of all of this is that social interaction in karate feels easy to me. Out in the real world, there are entire magazines dedicated to fashion and style. But at the dojo, if my outfit is clean and I'm shaven and shorn, I'm good. While consideration of bodily hygiene and other issues connected to exercise is an important courtesy, there are times people go so overboard they inhibit their training experiences and that of others. It is difficult to train well on a full stomach, but skipping a meal entirely results in diminished energy and dragon-breath. A good shower is normally a sufficient precaution against personal odors, even foot odor. The countless products available to combat every olfactory offense our bodies can produce are often perfumed overkill. Choose them carefully, with the understanding that your training partners often consider these cures to be worse than the malady.

Most of all, treat yourself well when preparing for class. A small portion of complex carbohydrates with plenty of water an hour prior to training is perfect. Use the bathroom before class so you don't have to miss any of the lesson or interrupt it to ask to be excused. And allow yourself plenty of time to arrive, dress, and self-train on the dojo floor before class. You're working hard to develop yourself. Honor that effort.

We are here to awaken from the illusion of our separateness.

Thich Nhat Hanh

BOWING

There is no other gesture I know that better indicates respect than a bow. It is a movement so beautiful that it transcends barriers of language and culture just as much as a smile. Many science fiction films, introducing characters with limbs unsuited for a physical exchange, communicate their courtesy with a bow. The bow is pure respect.

And it is no more than that. Karate is not a religion, and karate practitioners are not members of some cult. Contrary to the voiced concerns I occasionally encounter, bowing—whether to nothing, to an object, to a photograph, or to a person—does not have religious significance and should not impinge on your present spiritual beliefs. (In fact, and in contrast to common expectation, there are many more similarities between Eastern and Western religions than there are differences.[2])

The act of bowing might have a strong presence in Buddhism, but that doesn't make it a solely Buddhist act any more than an act of kneeling prior to an American pro-football game makes kneeling a Christian act. Simply put, he who bows defers to the universe in humility, understanding that he is but a part of it and seeking to be the best part he can be. By bowing to a photograph of an ancestor or teacher, he gives honor and thanks, recognizing the teacher as an inextricable part of himself. He does the same when he bows to you.

There is a process to a correct bow that is too often ignored, particularly by we Westerners in our haste to get to the next item on our agendas. Proper bowing is an opportunity for contemplation. It offers a chance to know that happiness has been found, here and now, in the presence of that to which you bow. Don't just toss off a quick nod. Instead, make *musubi dachi,* which is one of the *shizen tai* stances.[3] Your heels are together, your feet apart, to the extent that they are perpendicular. Your toes grab the floor. Your knees are straight but, as always, unlocked. Your hands are open with fingers aligned in

2 Thich Nhat Hanh, *Living Buddha, Living Christ* (New York, NY: Riverhead Books, 1995).

3 See chapter 4.

the *shuto* position,[4] but relaxed and placed comfortably at the sides of your thighs. Bend at the waist, and only the waist, keeping your spine straight. The deeper you bow, the more respect you show.

Breathing is incorporated as an element of the optimal bow.[5] Inhale throughout your steady descent, bending all the way until your upper body is at a 45-degree angle. Remain there as you exhale, with your eyes on your counterpart's feet. Inhale again as you deliberately rise with speed equal to your bow. This timing fully enables composure of your thoughts and also communicates your respect for others. In return for such mindful bowing, you will be rewarded with a sense of humility and meditative peace.

Karate always begins and ends with a bow.

Master Gichin Funakoshi

---

4 See chapter 5.

5 As illustrated by Masaaki Ueki, Senior Managing Director, Japan Karate Association, during the June, 2007 ISKF Master Camp, Green Lane, Pennsylvania.

THE DOJO FLOOR

The training area, or "dojo floor," is a special place indeed. If it's like the one at our school, it was hand-built by dedicated students specifically for the purpose of karate training. There's no place in your life quite like it.

The training deck itself is traditionally composed of varnished hardwood, but I have trained on surfaces of every conceivable material: tatami matting, tile, linoleum, plywood, parquet, concrete, asphalt, carpet, grass, and vinyl-coated, high-density foam matting (the choice for the Olympic Games, and what I use in my dojo). You may train in a dojo that might seem like it's not up to par with what you expected a dojo to be. It may be located in a multi-use facility, such as a YMCA basketball court or a church basement. Such a dojo is no less special than the most sequestered mountain training hall. Think about the assembled decades of knowledge you'll have access to, brought to you by your seniors, who gleaned it from their forebears. For these reasons and many more, the training area is to be treated as sacred space.

Sir Isaac Newton once said that if he had achieved much, it had been "by standing on the shoulders of giants." We will excel to the extent that we keep this in mind. At the front of a traditional dojo there will be a photograph or painting of Gichin Funakoshi, whom we honor as the father of our system of karate. Also (in the United States), there will usually be an American flag and a Japanese flag harmoniously hung on either side of the picture. The Japanese term for this area is *shomen*. These items are positioned to keep us mindful of, and grateful for, the efforts of those who developed the art we enjoy. In a multi-use facility, or outdoors where it is impractical to hang such reminders, it is still important to use the entrance to your training area as an opportunity to offer respect in this way. Whether it's a clear entry-point onto a purpose-built training floor, a swinging door into a gym, or a patch of grass, there should be a designated entrance into your training space. Here is where you must stop, face shomen, and bow before entering.

Contemplate the importance of this moment. It is an opportunity for you to be worthy of the inestimable efforts of your teachers and of those whose work has created the facility you are about to enjoy. It is a moment of peace, letting you clear your mind of the day's concerns and focus on the here and now. And bending over deeply invites the humility that will let you maximize your learning during your training period. So enjoy this moment. Bow slowly. Then enter this place that has been custom made for your training.

> ### Self-Training
>
> *After making musubi dachi, inhale deeply as you lean forward. Stay at the bottom of your bow for the full time it takes you to exhale. Then, inhale again as you come up. This three-part sequence provides many advantages. It keeps your back straight. It sets a pace that shows deep respect and enables mindfulness of that to which you bow. And it enriches your body with oxygen. As your bow ends, you will find yourself acutely awake to the recipient of your courtesy.*

So you've managed to make it onto the dojo floor, uniformed and ready to train. What do you do while you're waiting for class to begin? For one thing, you're likely to hear the clarion cry, "Rags!" which brings the opportunity to enjoy happy dojo maintenance with your friends. (If you don't know what this means, you'll soon discover why the dojo floor is always so clean!) In addition, there will be skills to hone and, invariably, friends to greet. In fact, you should maximize the time you have prior to class. Make every effort to arrive as early as possible, no later than fifteen minutes before class, and even earlier to allow time to change clothes and use the restroom if necessary. This will honor the time it takes to chat with the good friends that hard training always creates. Most importantly, you want to get on the floor early to stretch more than class time affords. This is of particular value in preventing injury and morning stiffness for those in their mid-thirties and older. You'll also want to rehearse techniques learned during prior classes. Karate skills accumulate and build in the way math or music skills do. You want to be as comfortable as possible with any particular section of training before you move on. Before class is good rehearsal time. Finally, be sure to hydrate. During very long classes there may be a break and a chance to drink fluids, but in a traditional class, the need to be completely focused requires that we train without interruption. Drink more water than you think you'll need—there won't be an opportunity to drink during class unless Sensei allows it for everyone, which will be rare. After you're sure all of your needs are met prior to the beginning of class, find a corner and focus on stretching or training.

Soon you'll hear a *senpai* (senior class member) shout, "Line up!" This means Sensei has arrived on the dojo floor and wishes to begin class. You'll find that your senpai will be sensitive to creating an environment supportive of Sensei's teaching intentions. This is because, for many years, he has worked on maximizing the time offered to him by Sensei. He has trained hard at the very concept of learning and has found that positioning himself quickly enables more learning to occur. As the senpai's rank increases, so will his sensitivity and, naturally, his responsibilities on the dojo floor. You are encouraged to emulate his example. If Sensei says to change position from one side of the dojo to another for reasons known only to Sensei in that moment, you will be hard pressed to get to your position faster than a senior class member gets to his. Try anyway. Respect your senpai. Don't hold up his learning process. When you hear the command to line up, don't meander. Run to your spot so your instruction can commence sooner.

CLASS STRUCTURE

Right away you will observe the astonishing attention to regimented detail pervasive in a traditional Japanese martial arts school of any sort. In my time of practicing these rituals, I've come to understand the benefits such extreme self-control offers, not only in the dojo but in the other areas of my life as well. I am far more aware of the placement of every part of my body—as well as the character of my words, my thoughts, and my actions—than I ever would be if I didn't allow myself the recurrent, private, and dedicated focus that Shotokan requires. Whether on the dojo floor, in a tournament, in a demonstration, or in your own back yard, these traditions facilitate physical and spiritual awareness beyond anything you've thought yourself capable. With focus and dedication, you'll find your natural strength and flexibility. There are moments in karate where you'll feel limitless. So enjoy the following traditions. Know that they are valid as areas of study and practice in and of themselves. They are doorways to a higher level of being.

Preliminary to the traditional Shotokan class, all students will line up in order according to rank, shoulder to shoulder, in a neat row facing shomen. In some schools, Black Belts form a line adjacent to the main line. The senior karateka in the main line will issue the following commands:

"Seiza!"

This is the command to kneel. Your left knee touches the floor first, your right knee is still up, pointing to your right. (This is because of the design of your gi, which crosses left over right. If you kneel with your right knee first, your gi opens up. I remember when, in an early class with Sensei Okazaki, he explained how in feudal Japan, a courier whose documents fell out of his gi would soon find his head falling off of his shoulders!) Next, bring your right knee to the ground. If a man puts two fists between his knees, they're about the right distance apart. Ladies' knees should be about one fist apart. Uncurl your toes so you are resting on the tops of your feet. You may let your feet be side by side, or you may cross one big toe over the other. Then allow your bottom to rest on your calves. We are unaccustomed to this position in the West, where our knees are seldom called upon to bend more than is necessary to sit in a chair. Your ankles may hurt. Let your conscious mind come away from your ankles, sit back, and allow your spine to align vertically. You will soon see that it is as if you carry a perfectly designed ergonomic chair with you at all times. When I sit in *seiza* I feel simultaneously alert and at rest. Place your hands at the tops of your thighs. Breathe. If your ankles hurt, I encourage you to go all the way into seiza for a few moments. Next time, try to remain there a moment longer, and the following time, a moment longer still. Your pain will go away with such practice, and you'll enjoy the flexibility and clarity of mind that millions of people do by regularly going into seiza.

Soon you'll hear the second command...

"MOKUSO!"

Meditate

It was only in the latter half of 2007, after twenty-seven years of karate training and after a privileged week of silence in the company of the venerable Thich Nhat Hanh, that I finally came to the appreciation that of all we study in the dojo—stances, strikes, kicks, blocks, body shifting, and even such deeper work as *kime* and relaxation—*mokuso* is our most important practice. In fact, it is to the extent we can bring mokuso to the rest of our training that we will find personal excellence and spiritual consciousness in our karate.

Later books in this series will offer further insights into this daily practice. For now, consider "mokuso!" a command that asks only two things of you:

1. Close your eyes.
2. Hear your breath.

That's all there is to it! Mokuso is at once easier than rolling off of a log and a challenge worthy of a lifetime of study.

It is during mokuso that you undergo the true transition between the outside world and your karate experience. Consider how often we find it infeasible to maintain a repetitive practice that involves a commute and focused study; these difficulties are what keep us from pursuing many of the goals we imagine for ourselves. For you, it may be an intense work schedule, complex academic studies, or simply an internal resistance to granting yourself permission to spend time and money on an activity that seems to only benefit you, rather than your children or spouse. Nevertheless, the fact that you're reading this book tells me you've made the commitment to at least give this a go. Mokuso can go a long way toward helping you get there.

There are many techniques you can use to facilitate mokuso. You might envision a pond in a beautiful place, without a single ripple on its surface. You can imagine floating in outer space, in complete nothingness. Another technique is to visualize an object that is pleasant to you but does not particularly invoke deep meaning, like a plain tea cup or a dogwood tree. I prefer to come to my breath, to envelop it in my awareness, following each in-breath from its birth to its passing, then attending to each out-breath in the same way. When our minds wander, one of these can provide a concept that helps bring us back to the here and the now. They reliably help us find peace.

It is a mistake, however, to dwell on the purpose of mokuso. Ultimately the idea is to "do" nothing. Mokuso is a moment in which, for once in your day, you *stop* doing. All day you've been doing tasks, particularly mental ones like planning, learning, contemplating, worrying, debating. During mokuso you can take all of that (sometimes I visualize taking my day's activities, wrapping them in brown paper, and tying them with a string) and set it aside. By the time you hear, *"Makuso yame!"* (cease meditating), I hope you will have "emptied your cup," permitting yourself to become fully present in the here and in the now of today's dojo experience. By practicing this process, you will come to realize how precious this hour of karate practice is. You will feel gratitude for this gift you give yourself, for your good health, and for the encouragements of your teacher. It will empower you to push past the many challenges you will face as a karateka.

If I somehow found myself in a strange reality where I could only choose a single one of the many beneficial elements of my karate training, I'd choose mokuso. Due to my good fortune in having the capacity for kind speech, and living at a time and place of historically low violence, I've never had cause to strike anyone with intent to harm and likely never will. But I must use my mind every day. Understanding its workings and the capacity to keep it calm in the face of uncertainty is, to me, the greatest benefit of our practice. There is far more worth talking about here, and we will in future books. For now, it is time to open your eyes.

"Shomen Ni Rei!"

Everyone in the class, including the sensei for that class, is invited to bow to shomen. In doing so, we formally acknowledge that we, as karateka, are links in a chain that extends long before our time, all the way back to Master Funakoshi. You need only think for a moment to understand that this chain extends beyond you as well; the quality of your karate powerfully affects those around you, and your karate training now will affect those whom you have yet to influence, or perhaps even those you will never personally meet.

In its mechanics, you may think of this more formal bow as duplicating the standing bow, except from a kneeling position. Since falling on your face would be somewhat embarrassing in this context, place your hands flat on the floor in front of your knees, fingers together, thumbs relaxed. Then, bow your head toward them. Out

Self-Training

Sit down, right now, cross legged on the floor. If that is uncomfortable you might sit on a bench or chair with both feet flat on the floor. In any case, sit erect but relaxed. Close your eyes and feel your breath enter and exit through your nostrils. Breathe no more deeply than normal and focus on that breath. Thich Nhat Hanh told us it is a miracle to be alive; we should enjoy our breathing. When you are distracted by a sound or a thought, don't try to shut it out. Acknowledge its existence, compartmentalize it, and bring your conscious mind back to your breathing. After a full minute, open your eyes.

If, in that minute, you were able to be truly present for your breathing even for a few seconds, take note. You've glimpsed what compels millions of practitioners like me toward a lifetime of meditation study.

Rei in Seiza

of courtesy to those behind you, keep your bottom down, seated on your folded legs, as best you can. Remain for the exhalation of your breath, then come up and resume your seiza, with your back straight and your hands resting on your thighs once again.

After Sensei spins about and faces the class, you'll hear...

"Sensei Ni Rei!"

Bow again in the same fashion, in acknowledgment of your respect for your sensei and your intention to follow his instructions without question. You must understand that no traditional dojo operates in the manner of a Western classroom. It is considered impertinent to raise a hand and bring attention to the issue of an individual. If questions are welcome, your sensei will tell you. Otherwise, simply do your best to follow along as best you can. This gives you the opportunity to struggle within yourself for answers, as those found within are always the most effective. After class, there are many opportunities to ask questions. Martial arts and other traditional Asian disciplines have been taught in this way for a very long time. The meditative quality of these methods of teaching is a large part of their allure to us Westerners. We must do our best to benefit from this method.

Warming Up

After bowing to Sensei, the class will commence, often with some words from Sensei, followed by a warm-up from a senpai. When this occurs, simply make your best effort to mimic the senpai's movements, holding any questions for after class. It is an important time;

your body becomes prepared for the exertions soon to come. A good warm-up will make it less likely that you will suffer an injury. Soon, Sensei will take over again, leading you through many of the activities described in this book, and much more than can be described in any book. At the end of class, Sensei may call a senpai up to the front again to conduct a warm-down. I enjoy warm-downs very much, especially when they are conducted in silence. I can introspectively focus on my flexibility.

Afterward, all students will be commanded to return to seiza for the closing ceremony, which involves the exact same process that began the class. There is an important addition, however. After mokuso has ended, you will hear the command...

"DOJO KUN!"

Training Hall Promise

The ethics stated in the *Dojo Kun* are inseparable from our decision to study karate. They constitute a critical part of our training. During his chairmanship of the International Shotokan Karate Federation, nearly every time there was a gathering of instructors, Shihan Teruyuki Okazaki emphasized the federation's duty to bring peace to the world. "If we live by Master Funakoshi's principles," he once said, "everything about our lives will fall into place." It is for this reason that Master Okazaki insisted on the use of the Dojo Kun in all ISKF dojos. Similarly, other federation chairs promulgate these same principles in thousands of karate schools worldwide, and they are heard in unaffiliated dojos as well.

You will hear a senior student speak the first line of the Dojo Kun. After she does, you will be swept along as it is spiritedly repeated by every student present. Do not rush its annunciation. If you take care to learn each unfamiliar syllable, you will soon find that it brings a comfortable close to a challenging class. Then, in many American schools like mine, the Dojo Kun is stated in English as well.

Dojo Kun:

Hitotsu! Jinkaku kansei ni tsutomuru koto!
Hitotsu! Makoto no michi o mamoru koto!
Hitotsu! Doryoku no seichin o yashinau koto!
Hitotsu! Reigi o omonzuru koto!
Hitotsu! Kekki no yu o imashimuru koto!

一、人格完成に努むること
一、誠の道を守ること
一、努力の精神を養うこと
一、礼儀を重んずること
一、血気の勇を戒むること

道場訓

Dojo Kun calligraphy by Master Teruyuki Okazaki

In English:
Seek perfection of character!
Be faithful!
Endeavor to excel!
Respect others!
Refrain from violent behavior!

Anyone would agree that these are sound principles to live by, whether one practices martial arts or not. It is vital, however, that fighting arts are practiced within a principled framework. Only then can we strive toward the excellence that is the promise of diligent training.

"Hitotsu!" (pronounced "Shtōts!") translates as "One thing!" This indicates the equal importance of each of these principles. By repeating these promises after each training, they will become embedded in your psyche enough to influence your behavior. Also, you will discover layers of meaning in each line of the Dojo Kun as you advance in your awareness of this art and in the subsequent awareness of yourself.

ARRIVING LATE

If you arrive after the moment class commences, you attend at the discretion of the instructor. The etiquette of entrance onto a dojo floor changes slightly in this circumstance, and reasonably so: this individual has taken the time to assemble a presentation to benefit *you*. The least you could do is show up for it! I once had a college professor whose door would slam like a portcullis—or perhaps more like a guillotine—precisely at the designated class start time. You couldn't get in even if you were held up by a car accident.

I have a different attitude for my own classes. I want my students there as much as they possibly can be. An adult student once told me why he missed a prior class. He explained the complexities of his household and described how the universe conspired to make it so he would have been late before he even got out the door. He decided it would be better not to come at all. I challenged his dedication to his karate. I described how I appreciate the frustration and embarrassment created by such times. "But," I said, "those events had already happened. You had already cost yourself several minutes of class. Even if you had shown up forty-five minutes late, you would have had fifteen minutes of training. Why throw them away?" I understand that most of my students are high achievers in the rest of their lives. Occasional delays are inevitable. When in doubt, show up anyway.

When you are late, it is appropriate to take care of all of your needs away from the dojo floor entrance. Take extra moments to make sure your gi is tied correctly, you've removed your jewelry, you've used the bathroom, and you've drunk plenty of water. There's nothing more flustering than hurrying out onto the floor, then having to excuse yourself *again* for something you hadn't thought of. Then, take a few extra *minutes* (not just a few seconds) to warm up. Find an out-of-the-way corner, perhaps in the dressing room, to do some quick calisthenics and stretching of your hamstrings, quads, abs, back, chest, arms, and neck. Hurrying into a class just to get injured will crimp your training far more than tardiness.

Then, when you are ready, take a musubi dachi stance at the dojo floor entrance.[6] You wait there for reasons of respect and safety; you should be humbly apologetic, anxious to learn, and reluctant to cause distraction to either the teacher or, worse, to a student needing to block at the same moment as your distraction! Keep your eyes focused on the instructor and wait for him or her to notice you. Chances are he already has. If more than a few moments go by, kneel in seiza. This is a visible indication of your willingness to wait and watch, for the rest of the class if necessary. When Sensei motions you forward, say nothing. Simply bow and run to your spot, always passing behind all other classmates, especially those senior to you in rank. This same strategy should be

---

6 See chapter 4.

used if you're not participating in the class but need to cross the floor during a class for some reason; this is obviously a situation to avoid if you can, but necessary in some dojos to get to the dressing room or bathroom.

THE ZEN OF GIVING SERVICE

All you've read prior to this point has been simply to guide you through the gateway that leads to your experience with the martial arts. Perhaps you've already realized that these guidelines apply metaphorically to gateways in many areas of your life.

There was a time in my early adulthood when I thought I understood my place as an American consumer. I thought that if I blessed a business with my patronage, I'd pay my money—as little of it as possible—and receive my goods or services in perfect condition. This seemed so logical that I'd grow frustrated when a merchant's performance was less than I expected. I remain a cost-conscious consumer, but now I understand that the "You Get What You Pay For" story runs more deeply than what can be measured by my ledger book.

Would you expect the same dining experience from two completely different types of restaurant? Imagine the difference between a family-run trattoria and a large, fast-food chain. The latter, brilliantly designed to reduce our cash and add to our fat stores at dizzying speed, requires minimal etiquette since it is run with uniform, semi-impersonal, robotic efficiency. An intimate bistro with six tables, however, seems to slow down both our world and our cares about it. I find myself far more patient there. I would't hesitate to assist the matron struggling with a serving tray piled with pasta, later tipping her based more on intent than completed service, even while paying triple what I would at a Wendy's, and all the while considering it a vastly superior experience. The trattoria slows me down enough to gain an understanding I wouldn't have had forty years ago: it is I who help make the experience superior. In that instance, I did so with my attitude of giving service toward Strega Nona in her struggles. This is the Zen of dining out.

I learned this lesson in a dojo. I was told early on, as all beginning students were, that it was my personal responsibility to keep the dojo clean. The floor was to be swept before every class. If I didn't see anyone else doing it, I was to take it upon myself to get the dust mop and sweep the floor. I was paying to be there, but I took great pleasure in hustling to keep it clean. If I saw a senpai sweeping or cleaning the floor—or cleaning anything else, for that matter—I felt it my duty to insist on grabbing the broom handle from him or her and taking over. If they said, "That's okay," I'd bow, describe the squat kicks Sensei would otherwise have me doing, and insist again. It was Zen and the Art of Dojo Maintenance.

It is, in fact, the Zen of everything. The more effort you put into the universe, the more the universe will give to you and those around you, unbidden. I encourage you to select areas of your life that are worth extra effort, and I further encourage you to consider your dojo a gymnasium for the exercise and development of your own attitude of giving service. This begins with paying your tuition happily, diligently, and always before it comes due. Then, taking it upon yourself to fix this fixture or to help with some administrative chore will bring benefits to you beyond the immediate completion of the task. (Unconsciously but invariably, the volunteers at my school seem to receive extra attention and time, and seem to form durable friendships with one another.) It will raise your esteem in the eyes of others and, through your very humility, will be leadership by example. You'll find potential for this throughout your dojo.

Another place for giving service is the acquisition of uniforms, books, equipment, and other accouterments of our art. You could likely purchase a given book or uniform less expensively elsewhere than if you bought it through your sensei. Even the largest martial arts schools, with students numbering in the thousands, have inferior purchasing power compared to internet companies and would be hard pressed to provide you with the best price. But those extra dollars go directly to bolstering the establishment from which you derive so much. The facilities and people associated with your greatest passion deserve abundant generosity, not frugality.

In conclusion, I invite you to do all you can to support your karate school. Remember also to have an attitude of giving service anywhere else you find great reward: your family, learning institutions, spiritual centers, or close friends. Choose carefully where you will direct you energies, then jump in with both feet and an open heart. Your reward will be a rich life.

DOJO ETIQUETTE GUIDE

Etiquette is prerequisite to learning. Commit to its mastery.

BEFORE ARRIVAL AT THE DOJO

❖ Practice good personal hygiene. Be clean and odor-free.

❖ Keep fingernails and toenails trimmed.

❖ Clean your gi.

AT THE DOJO, BEFORE CLASS BEGINS

❖ Remove your shoes.

❖ Register your attendance.

❖ Change quickly. Remove all jewelry. Restrict long hair.

❖ Be in uniform and ready to train at least ten minutes early.

❖ Bow to shomen upon entering or exiting the dojo floor.

❖ Participate in cleaning and preparing the dojo for training.

DURING CLASS

❖ If given no instruction, remain in shizen tai (natural stance) with your eyes on your imaginary opponent or, if he is offering an explanation, on Sensei.

❖ Catch your mind when it wanders. Return to the clarity of the present moment.

❖ Keep silent throughout class unless asked to do otherwise.

❖ Move quickly when asked to. Run.

❖ Learn the Dojo Kun quickly and thoroughly.

❖ If you arrive late, wait respectfully to be invited into class.

❖ Seek every opportunity to contribute to the organization and maintenance of your dojo.

Chapter 3

Basic Techniques

Before you are through being a White Belt, you will already be required to have competence in four stances, four blocking techniques, six strikes, and four front kick variations. There will be moments when this eighteen-item checklist will seem like an overwhelming amount of material to swallow in a very short period of time. There are, however, a few key qualitative generalizations to be made about virtually all techniques. As you enjoy class training in *kihon* (technical fundamentals), you'll want to continually check the following seven preliminary items to ensure they are driven deeply into your muscle memory. Your ability to grasp them will make it easier to develop effective karate. They are presented in the order in which most students are able to develop awareness of them, *not* in order of their importance. For now you should consider them equally important, which is why they're not numbered.

SEVEN ASPECTS OF KIHON

❖ The physical aspect of your karate always begins with your **stance**. Of these seven, it is the one aspect that will most determine the effectiveness of your technique, so be attentive to the details presented in the chapter devoted to this subject.

❖ Next is the chosen **technique**. Even if it feels strange or ineffective to you at first, make no assumptions as your sensei or senpai shows you how to perform a new move. Be a blank slate, and learn properly from the start.

❖ **Half-face** or **straight-face**—you'll hear one of these terms constantly as you learn to orient your body for the proper application of defense or offense, respectively. Rotating into a half-faced position draws your vital organs away from your attacker, brings increased power to the blocking technique, and prepares you kinesiologically for the delivery of a powerful counterattack. Rotating into a straight-faced position enables maximum concentration of power. It is important that your stance places your feet at hip's width, as described earlier, so your hip has adequate range to easily rotate between straight-face and half-face.

❖ The **draw hand**, or *hikite*—that is, the opposing hand from the technique hand, drawn to the hip as the basic strike or block is deployed. This is the aspect of technique most often overlooked by beginning students. What senior students understand, however, is that virtually all techniques make use of the entire body and are expressed with both hands. An improper draw hand robs much of the power from the technique being applied by the other hand. Indeed, your draw hand should be snapped back with exactly the same energy that is applied to the technique itself. With your elbow remaining close to the body, your fist draws back, fully rotated, ending just above your belt. When in a half-face position, strive for your forearm to end perpendicular to your line of travel.

❖ Regardless of the position of your body, it is important to keep your **head forward**. The generation of power promised by Shotokan karate requires relaxation in the parts of the body not being used. Keeping your head relaxed (inside and out!) can save your life. You'll hear, "Look first!" when you turn from one direction to another, and you must be relaxed to observe a threat as quickly as possible. This behavior is seen when a cat stalks its prey. Regardless of the movement of its body, its head remains steady, enabling it to take full advantage of its stereoscopic vision by keeping both eyes equidistant from its target. You must do this as well.

❖ Your capacity to keep your gaze on your **opponent's eyes** could make the difference between surviving an attack and being overcome by one. Many of us find it hard to look steadily into another person's eyes, which can be uncomfortable. But in my dojo we practice it and overcome that discomfort as we develop this vital skill. Master Hirokazu Kanazawa described it as necessary for knowing what your opponent will do in a fight before he does it. Through your opponent's eyes, Kanazawa said, you learn to become his mirror and therefore come to see that he is not your antagonist at all—an empowering concept. When you face a partner, the best method is to simply look at his eyes without thought. This best enables you to see who that person truly is and communicates your stead-fastness to him. If that makes you feel uncomfortable, start with one eye or the other, or simply focus on the bridge of his nose. Always practice this gaze in your mind when you face forward in class and, whenever possible, when you look into the eyes of an opponent.

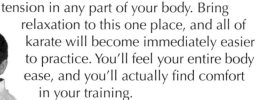

Self-Training

Here's a reliable way to discover which of the "corners" of your feet takes more weight than it should. Tape a few sections of 1/2" bubble wrap to the floor. Rather than doing what you want to do, try walking across it, slowly, striving to not pop a single bubble. Only by balancing your weight across each foot can you achieve this as you step.

❖ Often, the last thing beginning karateka accomplish in their initial development is to get their **shoulders relaxed.** Relaxation is absolutely fundamental to self-defense and to the generation of power. Hunched shoulders are normally the first indicator that you are too tense, but watch for tension in any part of your body. Bring relaxation to this one place, and all of karate will become immediately easier to practice. You'll feel your entire body ease, and you'll actually find comfort in your training.

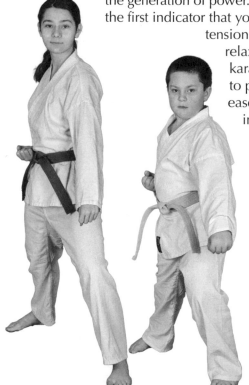

Chapter 4

Stances

SHIZEN TAI

Natural Stance

Stand up, right now.

Breathe in.

Breathe out.

Relax.

There: you probably situated yourself into something a non-martial artist would call a normal standing position. We call it *shizen tai*, or "natural stance." Shizen tai is actually a category of stances and, as such, it is perhaps the most important of stance categories since it is where we spend most of our time. Unless you're more comfortable in an outward-tension horse stance while waiting in line at Starbucks, chances are you're waiting there in something close to a variation of shizen tai.

There is more to it than this, of course. You'll be told to revert to shizen tai following one challenging drill or another, just when you're sucking wind and feeling sorry for yourself. The mistake, then, is to consider the command of "shizen tai!" as permission to be absent-mindedly "at ease." Quite the opposite; I tell my students to consider shizen tai as "standing on purpose."

The common thread of a proper shizen tai stance is that you are wide awake and ready, with expanded senses, loose joints, and proper body alignment. We'll touch on each of these points in reverse order.

BODY ALIGNMENT — Let's conduct a self-study, starting where our bodies begin: at the ground. You should feel all four corners of your feet carrying equal weight.[7] Consider a table: it is not optimally stable until the weight its four legs share is balanced. Similarly, you will soon see it is impossible for your body to be in balance if your feet aren't first. Invariably, we've gained a habit of putting additional pressure on one of the corners of our feet. A good martial artist can think of himself as standing on eight equal points. This is part of the reason such solid balance can be found while standing on one foot.

Your pelvis and spine should similarly be freed and centered in their own equilibrium. Your body becomes more efficiently aligned if you tuck your pelvis slightly under your torso.

Next come your shoulders and arms. Here is a method for finding the best resting place for them. Stand in a relaxed but alert fashion. Push your shoulders all the way forward and hold them there for a moment. Then pull them all the way back, as though to touch your shoulder blades together. Move them like this, fully forward, then fully back. When you've got a feel for their range, bring your shoulders to their natural center point. Your shoulder structure should drape comfortably over your rib cage, starting from your trapezius and clavicle and ending with your deltoids wrapping over the tops of your arms. This brief practice lets you gain a conscious sense of where your shoulders *want* to be.

Include your neck and head in this self-study. Your cervical spine enters the base of your skull, providing a perfect pivot point for your eight-pound head. Rotating your head side to side and back and forth slightly, you'll become aware of this attachment point right between your earlobes, and you'll enjoy an immediate sense of conscious balance.

---

7 As practiced in the Bubble Wrap exercise in chapter 3.

LOOSE JOINTS — Take the time to bring conscious control to each of the primary joints required for standing: your knees, pelvis, shoulders, and neck. These joints, especially your knees, should be straight but not locked or hyper-extended. As above, experiment with the exact positioning of each of them, playing with their range of motion and settling on the midpoint dictated by each joint's comfortable positioning.

EXPANDED SENSES — As expressed above, we practice an attitude of self-defense 100 percent of the time we are on the dojo floor. Shizen tai is the place for us to begin this practice.

Find a spot on the wall at eye level. It is impossible to focus on all spots in the room, but it is possible to have the discipline to focus on just one. Then, by use of your peripheral vision, you can observe everything else happening in the room. By isolating the one spot, the others become perceptible.

You can even train your peripheral vision to gain greater sensitivity than it currently possesses. Various exercises can develop your speed in perceiving spots on the wall as you turn, or for expanding your field of view, or for maintaining your perceptive ability under duress. All of these are worthwhile and will be studied in your karate practice. Their development might be necessary to cope with a life-threatening situation one day. And, short of such a need, their development will lead to a more robust living experience in your peaceful daily life.

With practice, it will only take you a moment each day to do this body scan, but the benefits of it are remarkable. Those of us who stand for lectures, meetings, or in lines may have developed a habit of locking our joints so our weight can be mindlessly supported by our frame. In fact, this is much more of a strain and leads to that exhausted feeling your bones have when you flop into a seat after waiting for public transportation. By contrast, shizen tai brings a feeling of being able to move quickly in any direction you need to. It can and should be consciously practiced in any of these circumstances until you develop the muscle memory that enables it to become a positive habit. You will be able to stand in shizen tai, tirelessly, all day.

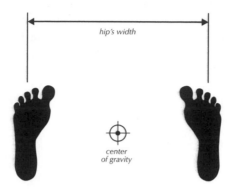

hip's width

center
of gravity

HEIKO DACHI

Parallel Stance

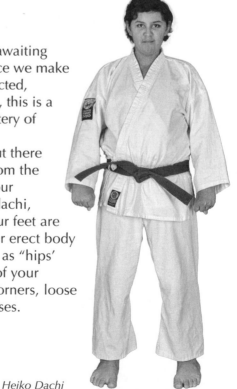

This is the stance we make while awaiting Sensei's instructions. It is also the stance we make while ascertaining whether an unexpected, hostile encounter is a threat. Therefore, this is a stance worth training toward. The mastery of this stance may save your life.

Heiko dachi may seem simple, but there is much to it. Imagine a line drawn from the center of your heel to the center of your middle toe. When standing in heiko dachi, these lines must be parallel, while your feet are separated just enough to stabilize your erect body —what your sensei will likely refer to as "hips' width" apart. From there, all aspects of your natural stance must be correct: foot corners, loose joints, body alignment, expanded senses.

Heiko Dachi

Standing on purpose like this has many benefits. Have you ever spent just a couple of hours at a mall and come home exhausted? I'll bet you spent much or all of your time with your knees and other joints locked and your body out of alignment. Someone with a good understanding of heiko dachi, however, can tirelessly stand all day. And, specifically with regard to karate, competence in this stance will determine your ability to fluidly and quickly take action.

MUSUBI DACHI

Knot Stance

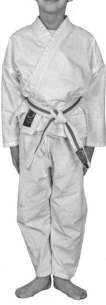

This is the stance we use to show our willingness to bow, and it is the stance we bow from. But its capacity to protect our femoral arteries, its side-knee support, and its foot positioning for angular kicks give musubi dachi self-defense value as well.

Position your heels so they are touching. The center lines of your feet extend 45° in either direction from your line of sight, and 90° from each other. Grip the floor with your toes subtly but firmly. If you look down you can see how this stance received its name: your feet resemble the knot in your belt.

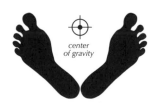

center
of gravity

Musubi Dachi

As with all stances, musubi dachi involves your entire body. Check your joints, alignment, senses, and breathing.

ZENKUTSU DACHI

Front Stance

Start in heiko dachi, and take a big step out with your left leg. Then, bend your front knee. You'll immediately feel like you're in a "front stance."

Next, and most importantly, make sure your back is straight. That is, tuck your pelvis under your head, shoulders, and properly curved spine. This may be impossible to imagine right now, but over time, front stance will actually become comfortable to you, your powerful legs feeling like able shock absorbers and strong pistons facilitating spectacular and effective techniques. Having a correct posture is necessary before this can ever become the case.

Position your feet so they are twice your shoulders' width apart at the heel. They also need to be hip's width apart on a line perpendicular

Zenkutsu Dachi

to your direction of travel, as shown in the
drawing on this page. Your front knee is
bent deeply, such that a plumb line hung
from it would touch directly in front of
your toes. Your back foot should be
rotated as far toward the front as
possible while keeping your heel on the
floor. Your front foot should be rotated
inward slightly, and your front knee should
be counter-rotated, but only slightly.
Excessive exterior torque can strain and, over
time, even injure complex knee structures.
Your goal is to build strength and stability.
Only rotate enough to create a solid grounding
with the floor and dynamic tension in your
stance. Finally, your center of gravity should rest 60
percent toward your front foot.

hip's width

center
of gravity

2x shoulders' width

Usually, by the time I've explained all of this to a
new student, his or her quadriceps are quivering to the
point where I have to tell them to stand back up—as soon
as they've gotten into the position! How could you possibly   do
karate from such a difficult stance? Be faithful. If you continue your
training, you will one day understand that this offensive stance is
perfectly designed to generate more power than you now believe
possible.

KOKUTSU DACHI

Back Stance

This time start in musubi dachi (the one you would use to bow to someone), and take that same big step out with your left leg until your heels are once again twice your shoulders' width apart. This time, however, your heels need to be on one line, rather than your hip's width apart as they were in *zenkutsu dachi*. For *kokutsu*, you might feel as if you are on a tightrope, but you'll soon find this to be a stable stance indeed.

While your heels align, the center lines of your feet should be perpendicular to one another. Bend your rear leg deeply, and create outward tension by rotating your knee slightly backward.

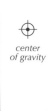

Your front knee should be bent as well—not as deeply as your rear leg, but just a little more than unlocked. Be sure your hips and torso are aligned so you are not leaning in any direction. And, as always, slightly grab the floor with the toes of both feet. You should feel like your legs are able shock absorbers. Try to sink comfortably in this stance, moving up and down lithely with the large muscles in your legs. Imagine yourself to be agile and capable of action in this stance.

You will be.

2x shoulders' width

⊕
center
of gravity

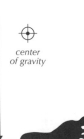

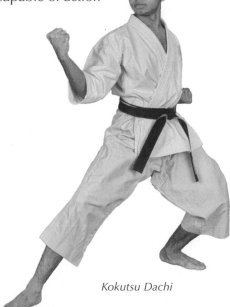

Kokutsu Dachi

Chapter 5

Blocking

Master Okazaki, in his instructor's training classes, frequently emphasized the *defensive* nature of karate-do, "the way of the empty hand." Accordingly, when teaching kihon, he encouraged us to teach our students defensive techniques before teaching punches, kicks, or strikes. That priority is reflected in this book, as it should be in your training. In karate, as in life, striking is much easier—and much less effective—than evading.

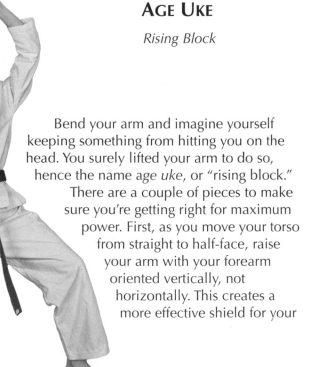

AGE UKE

Rising Block

Bend your arm and imagine yourself keeping something from hitting you on the head. You surely lifted your arm to do so, hence the name a*ge uke*, or "rising block." There are a couple of pieces to make sure you're getting right for maximum power. First, as you move your torso from straight to half-face, raise your arm with your forearm oriented vertically, not horizontally. This creates a more effective shield for your

Jodan Age Uke

chest, neck, and face as you put the block into place. Your elbow should remain close to your torso as you raise your arm. You should also have a tight fist as you do so, with the palm of your fist facing you. Then, at the last instant, rotate your wrist so your palm faces away from you. Your arm should be placed high enough that your opponent cannot see the top of your head above it. Your forearm should be one fist's width from the top of your head, and held at a 45° angle so that a downward blow would handily glance off of it.

CHUDAN SOTO UDE UKE

Mid-level Outside-to-Inside Block

To prepare for a mid-level block, bring one fist to your ear as though you are answering a desk telephone. Now rotate your fist so your knuckles face forward, your palm faces away from you, and your thumb is on the bottom of your fist. Move your elbow so it points somewhat behind your head.

To execute the block, rotate your torso to half-face and sweep your bent arm forward so it ends directly in front of you. At the last

Soto Ude Uke

moment, rotate your wrist. Your fist should be even with your shoulder, and your elbow should be one fist's width from your ribcage. Your arm has now formed a shield that can protect your entire midsection.

This is a potent defensive technique. I encourage you to spend a great amount of time developing it. At higher levels of training, you will discover many variations of *ude uke* that are effective in a variety of circumstances. In addition, after the block has been completed, your arm is ideally positioned to launch a variety of rapid counter attacks. Practice ude uke; it is the first step toward these exciting techniques.

BARAI UKE

Downward Sweeping Block

To prepare for a downward block, bring your fist across your chest to your opposite ear. Your elbow should be in front of your chest, and the palm of your fist must be rotated so it faces your ear.

Execution of the block is done by sweeping your arm downward and directly in front of you. Again, keep your elbow close to your torso and rotate your wrist at the last instant, when your arm nearly straightens (but does not lock). Your arm ends with your elbow one fist's width from your ribcage again. Whether you are in a front or back stance, your fist should remain one fist's width above your knee.

Gedan Barai Uke

SHUTO UKE

Knife-hand Block

Before you can use this uke technique, you must first be able to place your hand in *shuto* position. To do so, hold your palm flat and your four fingers straight and together. You should have the feeling that your index finger pushes toward your middle finger and your pinky finger pushes toward your ring finger. Your thumb bends and tucks neatly alongside your palm, not in front of it. Your entire hand, made of bone and muscle and having relatively little fat, should feel very solid, like a piece of steel. Finally, put a slight bend in the tips of your fingers, causing tension along your hand and forearm like the leaf spring in a car's suspension. Your hand should feel like a tempered knife. Indeed, your entire forearm should feel like a sword.

Now to *move* it like a sword. Similar to the preparatory move for barai, put your arm across your chest with your palm to your opposite ear, except this time your hand is held in shuto position. Strike with your arm diagonally in front of you, leading with your elbow, as demonstrated by your sensei or senpai. Rotate your wrist in the last instant of the movement, snapping your hand into a 45° angle. Your fingertips end at the level of your relaxed shoulder, and, similar to *chudan soto ude uke*, your elbow ends a fist's width from your ribcage. The elbow joint is held at a 90° angle.

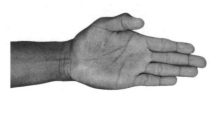

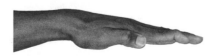

Shuto uke is most often practiced in *kokutsu dachi,* or back stance. When this is the case, your draw hand is performed somewhat differently during the motion of shuto uke than it is during most blocks, strikes, and punches. When you bring the palm of your striking hand up to your ear, extend the other hand straight out and palm down in front of you, holding it, too, in a shuto position. Your elbows should be crossed, your chest contracted. Then, expand your chest and draw your shoulder blades together. Simultaneous to performing the strike, sharply retract your draw hand, rotating it at the last instant into a position that protects your solar plexus. Again, one technique requires the use of both hands. Your draw hand performs double-duty, applying an elbow strike to the rear.

The pisiform bone creates the bump on the lower, proximal side of your palm (opposite your thumb). Indicating the relationship between the draw hand's pisiform and the solar plexus, I tell my students, "Put this bump in that dent." Your hand must remain in the shuto position with your palm facing up perfectly. You should now be able to balance a glass of water on that palm without spilling it!

Chapter 6

Striking

MAKING A FIST

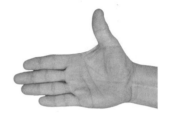

I love to box. In American boxing, I can jab, cross, and upper cut. I use the strength and weight of my arm — a little less than seven and a half pounds[8]—to execute techniques which, when I'm on my game, can rattle an opponent.

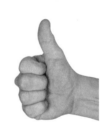

But I prefer karate. With Shotokan, I get to choose from many more weapons. Even when I use my hands alone, they're more effective: I grab the floor with my feet, relax my muscles, rotate, and then snap them all into a moment's tension, bringing the strength and weight of my entire body through my fist. I hit with 170 pounds, not seven and a half.

A punch, properly propelled by a competent Black Belt, can devastate. But my fist must be superbly prepared to be used in this fashion, or I'll cause more damage to myself than I will to whatever it is I'm hitting.

---

8 R. F. Chandler, *Investigation of Inertial Properties of the Human Body* (Ft. Belvoir Defense Technical Information Center, 1975). 72–79.

There are five steps to making a fist properly:

1. Extend your hand, with your fingers together and your thumb out.
2. Curl the tops of your fingers down and squeeze them into a bear paw. Your finger joints are severely curved, but the knuckles on the back of your hand are still straight. Squeeze your fingertips into the top of your palm as tightly as possible.
3. Roll your fingers down into your palm, keeping your fingers curled tight.
4. Wrap your thumb tightly around your bundled fingers.
5. At this point you may feel as if your fist is about to explode. Now, without backing off on your grip, relax your muscles. Keep your fingers in this position, just don't put any effort into it.

Self-Training

Try making a fist quickly, without going through the steps listed here. Push on the striking surface of your first two fingers. See how they collapse in? Now, carefully make your fist as shown, then push on your knuckles. They're far more stable, a heartier weapon. Rather than absorbing as much force as a looser fist would, your proper fist will transmit the energy into your target.

With practice, this will become easy for you to do, even comforting, the way a seat belt becomes reassuring in a car—a proper fist will be so familiar that *not* making one will seem out of the question.

Watch what Black Belts do with their fists when they go into shizen tai. You'll catch them in the long-time habit of making their fists carefully every time they enter a natural stance. Make sure you cultivate this habit, too.

Self-Training

Practice choku tzuki at home in the fist-exchanging manner described. After ten repetitions, increase your speed, but only slightly. An onlooker would still think you're moving very slowly. Don't get bored; doing it in this way will pay big dividends later. After ten reps at this speed, increase it slightly again. After one hundred reps, you'll be snapping your fists quickly. When practicing any karate technique, always be sure you define moving at speed as going as fast as possible while still doing the motion correctly.

CHOKU TZUKI

Straight Punch

Standing in a proper shizen tai, like heiko dachi,[9] simply place one fist in front of you, palm down. As is the case with blocking, bring your draw hand back to an upside down position above your belt. Direct your punching hand toward the center of the body of an imaginary opponent. Aim it exactly at the solar plexus of a nonexistent person of your own size who is standing opposite you. Your gaze should be on the eyes of this ethereal karateka. Like your other joints, your arm should be straight but not locked. Relax your shoulders. Imagine a drop of water placed on the shoulder of your punching arm would be able to run steadily down your arm to your fist.

Now, slowly, exchange your fists. As one extends, the other retracts. Always be as mindful of your draw hand as you are of your striking hand; don't just worry about hitting something. Exchange fists again. Continue punching in this balanced manner. Do it in a slow, rhythmic motion, firmly feeling the end of the movement in both arms with each repetition. After each punch, do a quick mental check of both fists to confirm that each is positioned properly. Remember to keep your shoulders relaxed. Let your upper arm swing off of your shoulder like a pendulum, your elbow staying close to your body, not coming away from it, during its path.

When punching—this goes for any of the methods described in this book—your elbow should always follow your fist, never rotating out of the path of your fist. Turn your fist over only at the very last instant. When it lands, imagine your punching hand

---

9 See chapter 4.

strikes only with the first two knuckles. Then, when you exchange hands, be sure the space previously occupied by the first two knuckles of the left hand is exactly the space occupied by the first two knuckles of the right hand.

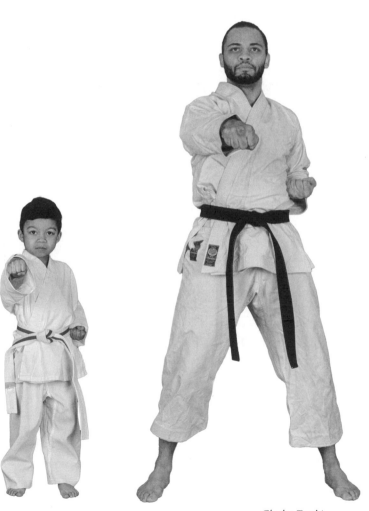

Choku Tzuki

GYAKU TZUKI

Reverse Punch

Now you will learn the punch you'll see relied upon most often in karate tournaments. By the time you are a Black Belt, this punch will happen so easily and with such force and power, you will understand the reason we all repeat Mr. Funakoshi's fifth Dojo Kun.

For *gyaku tzuki*, you'll stand in zenkutsu dachi.[10] Put your left foot forward as shown in the photo below. You'll like doing offensive techniques from a front stance, and you'll see that advanced Black Belts often prefer it for executing their most powerful punches, kicks, and strikes. While in front stance, punch as you did in choku tzuki: left sharp draw hand, shoulders relaxed, joints unlocked, punching toward your imaginary opponent's solar plexus with your right hand's first two knuckles. For this punch, you will always use the fist that is opposite your forward foot. It is this opposition that causes this straight-faced punch to be named as it is.

There's more to this punch than arm movement. In fact, you will come to understand your arm movement isn't even the most important aspect of generating power in your punch. This force comes from a concerted effort emanating from your hips and abdominal muscles. We'll discuss this in careful detail later. For now, when you punch with gyaku tzuki in zenkutsu

---

10 See chapter 4.

Gyaku Tzuki

dachi, understand that your hips must face forward while your pelvis remains tucked under your straight, vertical spine.

Self-Training

You can do your own "Night of 1,000 Punches" in a way that's easier than you might think. Simply get comfortable in your front stance. Flip your hips back and forth, counting to yourself. Work on your relaxation. Be sure your stance stays consistent, with outward tension on your knee as it remains over your toes. Use less and less energy to do the punches, striving to just flip your hip into straight and half-face. Start by counting to ten five times. That's one hundred punches! Then switch feet and do it again. Tomorrow, do more.

KEZAMI TZUKI

Jab Punch

Remaining in zenkutsu dachi, rotate your hips into a half-face position—unusual for an attack, as half-face positioning is most often associated with defense—and slowly let your left arm straighten into a jab. As it does so, your elbow follows your fist, your forearm remaining aligned in the path of the punch like the perfect flight of an arrow. The forearm of your draw hand, however, should be behind you, perpendicular to your line of attack, not unlike the draw hand for a block. In class drills, we typically punch *jodan* or face-level with our *kezami tzuki* and *chudan* or stomach level with our gyaku tzuki.[11] The important point is to develop the rotation of your hips between half- and straight-face. Your feet must be hips' width apart to facilitate this. Don't let your knee collapse when punching kezami tzuki.

Flip back and forth between pages 54 and 56 to enjoy the little animation of the gyaku tzuki/kezami tzuki punching drill. In our dojo, we sometimes have a "Night of 1,000 Punches." We all make front stance and flip between kezami tzuki and gyaku tzuki. I get the sequence started, correcting stances and technique as everyone

---

11 Addressed in detail under "Aiming" in chapter 9.

does one punch every time I count. Finally, I begin counting to ten in Japanese. At each count, we all do two punches, first kezami tzuki, then gyaku tzuki right away. After I count ten, the highest-ranking karateka immediately follows and counts ten, with the class merrily double-punching with each count. Then the next highest-ranking karateka counts ten, and so forth, until we've done ten times as many double punches as there are students in the class.

There is an intensity to this class, yes, but having survived more than my fair share of them, I've found there to be a wonderful, meditative quality to them, like Taiko, Native American, and African tribal drumming. It provides an opportunity to focus on my breathing and to clear my mind of my concerns. After all, if I allowed myself to think about how much my front leg's quadricep hurts, I wouldn't last very long. But as is the case with most things in karate, it's far more about my attitude than it is about my strength. I allow myself to become absorbed with the focal point that my eyes are fixed on. I work on relaxing more and more as the punches continue until I feel like my entire body knows what to do all by itself, flipping on its own hinge. I enjoy the athleticism and good health that enable me to do my karate.

When many people think of hand-to-hand fighting, their imagination is limited to fisticuffs. Karate is famous for using numerous parts of the body as weapons. While punches are technically strikes, there are strikes that can create damage in places that kicks and punches often cannot. You will learn two such techniques while you are a White Belt.

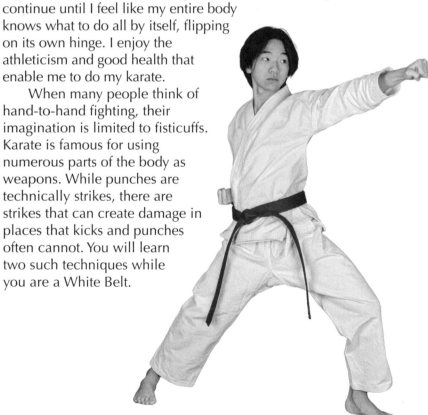

Kezami Tzuki

KENTSUI

Hammer Fist

When you make a fist properly, you will notice that the pinky side of the palm emerges and is tensed. It certainly looks, and swings, like a hammer. Used as a weapon driven by the underarm musculature of your triceps, latissimus dorsi and serratus anterior, *kentsui* makes for an incredibly strong blow to soft and even hard targets. As a vertical strike, it is effective against the collar bone, shoulder, nose, cheek bone, forehead, and crown. Used in a roundhouse fashion, it is effective against the temple, ear, jaw, neck, and ribs.

The vertical application of kentsui is learned during White Belt training. Make your tight fist, then raise your relaxed arm above your head. As you squeeze your core and underarm muscles, lead the swing of your fist with your elbow. It is vital to keep your arm relaxed as it descends. Unlike punching and blocking, there is no rotation of the fist with this technique.

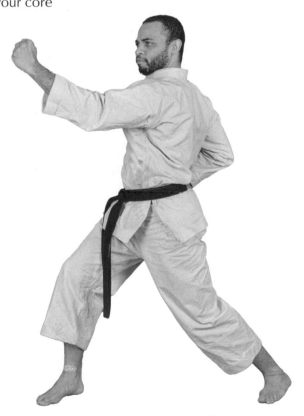

Kentsui

SHUTO UCHI

Knife-Hand Strike

When you become a competent Black Belt, *shuto uchi* will be a deadly component of your arsenal. Since you are using the edge of your palm, the striking surface is reduced from your fist, enabling you to apply greater force over the area you are striking.

Like kentsui, shuto uchi can be deployed in a vertical fashion by beginning over the head and striking downward. When using shuto uchi in a horizontal fashion, bring the back of your right hand up to your right ear, fingers forward and elbow back like you would for ude uke, except your hand is in shuto position. Strike horizontally to a target in front of you, rotating your wrist at the last instant so your palm is up. You can also strike in the other direction by bringing the palm of your shuto hand to your opposite ear, striking horizontally, and rotating at the last instant so your palm faces down. At the end of shuto uchi, the arm is straight but unlocked.

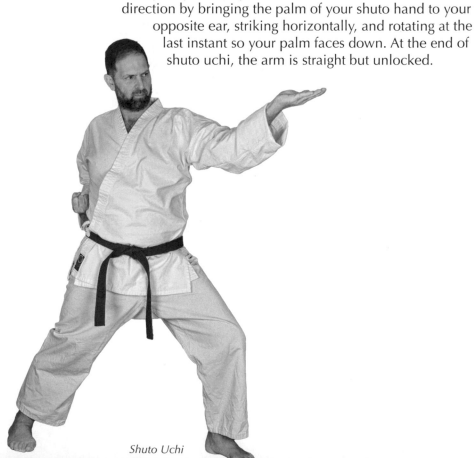

Shuto Uchi

Chapter 7

Kicking

If you've ever looked into the face of a monkey, as I have, I'm sure your shared ancestry became as immediately and overwhelmingly apparent to you as mine did to me. Unfortunately, not being simians means we have lost many of the advantages our monkey-cousins retain. We don't use our feet for eating, writing, washing, touching, and all of the other activities we are far more comfortable using our hands to perform. For this reason, you must work harder to train your legs to use them with precision.

You want your legs in your arsenal. They have four times the strength of your arms. They also enable farther-reaching attacks than do any other parts of your body. Your legs increase your range and let you defend yourself from a safer distance.

MAE GERI KEAGE

Front Snapping Kick

You would be hard pressed to find a frontal attack that is more linear from your body center than *mae geri*. It's a direct, logical, core motion. Nevertheless, most people are only familiar with the kind of kick performed in a game of soccer. Mae geri is much different than a sports kick.

The most important leg-related element of mae geri, or any kick, has to do with the leg you're *not* kicking with. Your capacity to grab the floor with your foot and develop a strong supporting leg will determine the power and stability of your kick. For this reason it is common for right-handed Black Belts to kick more effectively with their left leg, and vice versa.

Leg flexibility is another important element, though not for the reason you might think. True, you can only kick as high as your flexibility will allow, and since your most powerful kick is done short of the limit of your flexibility, it affects the height of an effective kick as well. But there are other ways to attack those targets. No, increased relaxation is the key benefit of flexibility, just as relaxation is prerequisite to the full generation of power. For thousands of years the practice of yoga has been used toward the cultivation of inner peace. This can also be cultivated in karate by fully surrendering to your senpai-led warm-up and warm-down stretches, and by finding the limits of your flexibility and lingering there during after-class stretching. As yogis know, the edge of a stretch is a most challenging place to relax. Another is while you're being attacked. Practicing karate teaches you to relax in the most stressful situation imaginable. It teaches you to relax anywhere.

As your ability to relax improves, so will your kick. Your body is made up of 40 percent leg. Nevertheless, in time, you'll be able to whip your legs as deftly as you can whip a towel.

The whipping action of mae geri keage begins with raising your knee toward your chest. This alone requires a good understanding of relaxation. Keep your upper body loose, your head level, your arms at your sides. Be sure to breathe comfortably when you practice. Your legs will be happier too as you enrich the blood flow to their thirsty muscles with oxygen. As you bring your knee up, curl up your toes, exposing the ball of your foot as the striking surface

* Knee Up
* Toes up
* Support leg bent
* Foot gripping the floor

Self-Training

Standing in shizen tai, pick up your knee. It should be high enough to balance a glass of water on your thigh. Hold it for a moment, then put it back down on purpose rather than just letting gravity take it. Pick up the other knee, hold it, put it back down. If you have trouble balancing, grip the floor with your other foot and bend the knee of your support leg a little.

Lift one leg again, this time feeling your knee come up with the contraction of your abdominal muscles as your forearm would when you contract your biceps.

Do this a few more times, now making sure your toes curl up.

During the next few reps, point your knee at a spot on a wall to represent the stomach of your imagined opponent. Like a gun sight, your foot will strike wherever your knee points.

Finally, be sure your upper body is relaxed throughout these motions. Don't bob your head.

Take plenty of time to develop this portion of your kick. Snapping your foot out and back is simple. It is here that the strength, control, and range of this devastating attack are forged.

and keeping the bottom of your foot level with the floor. It bears repeating: curl your toes up, not down! You'll use your most powerful muscles to send your tiny toe bones toward a blocking opponent; it's best to have them up and out of the way.

The next step may seem completely unintuitive: you must use your hips to kick! Imagine yourself not using your leg muscles at all. Thrust your hips forward. Allow your foot to lash out as a result of the momentum generated by your hips, like the tip of a wet towel would after your arm flicked it. Extend your foot, keeping the bottom of it as close to parallel with the floor as you can, curling your toes up. With your toes safely out of the way, strike with the ball of your foot. I've created another animation between these two photographs. Flip them back and forth to see what a proper kick motion looks like.

As suddenly as it was thrust forward, your pelvis should rock back into position, causing your leg to snap back quickly—so quickly that you could imagine kicking yourself in your hindquarters with your heel. This adds power to your kick and prevents your opponent from catching your foot. Continue the snap-back momentum by purposefully placing your foot back down on the floor. Never simply use gravity. Always reassert your stance in a minimum amount of time. You can use the animation to demonstrate this, too.

Mae geri keage is my favorite kick. Practicing it has kept sparring partners at bay, has scored points for me in tournaments, and has kept my knees lithe and lubricated as I've gotten old.

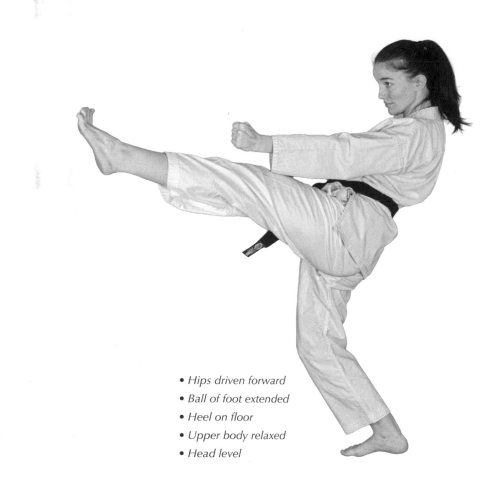

- *Hips driven forward*
- *Ball of foot extended*
- *Heel on floor*
- *Upper body relaxed*
- *Head level*

Chapter 8

Body Shifting

Should you ever need to actually defend yourself, chances are you won't be able to just stand in one place performing karate techniques! You'll need to shift your body in this direction or that, and your karate will need to be executed in harmony with your body movements. This is the practice of *tai sabaki*.

HIP ROTATION

Look back at the animation of gyaku tzuki and kezami tzuki that you get by flipping between pages 54 and 56. You'll notice the karateka's hips face forward to execute gyaku tzuki, but they face to the side when punching with kezami tzuki. This movement is fundamental to karate. The rotation of your hips, when understood, brings both speed and power to techniques and body shifts that simply can't be rivaled by the conventional body movements we Westerners have been raised with.

Each time you execute an upper body technique in front stance, whether it's a block, punch, or strike, your primary concern should be your awareness of your hip rotation and ending position. In time you will bring this awareness to your kicks and body shifts as well, regardless of your stance. For now, though, make careful note of when you're told to be in half-face or straight-face position. Generally speaking, blocking is done in half-face, attacks are executed with straight-face. There are exceptions, some of which you've already learned, like kezami tzuki and shuto uchi. The final word on facings is given by your sensei. Point the knot of your belt wherever he or she says, consistently.

One more point: look back at the stance diagram for zenkutsu dachi on page 40. You will notice the requirement that your feet are placed hips' width apart relative to the direction you are facing. Only in a stance so structured can you rotate your hips to the extent required for basic Shotokan techniques.

C-STEP

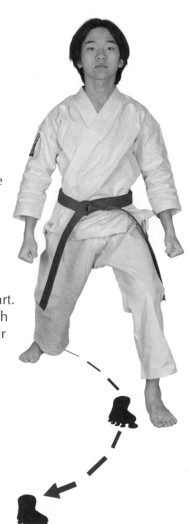

When shifting from one place to the next during the practical application of karate, it is helpful to utilize the C-Step. This enables you to move reliably to a stance that maintains the critical hips' width foot position.

Begin in zenkutsu dachi, with your feet properly placed one hip's width apart. Then drive your hips forward. Don't push off from your back foot. Rather, pull your rear leg to you from the momentum created by your forward-thrusting hips. Allow your feet to come together, then sweep your front foot out until it reaches a position two shoulders' length and one hip's width from your other foot. Land in a perfect front stance, with your front foot's toes rotated in slightly while you hold outward tension on your front knee.

During C-Step, your stepping foot must remain close to the floor—one paper's thickness, as we say. This minimal distance lets you more quickly adjust to an unexpected need to change directions or tactics. Also important is keeping your head and upper body at the same level as you travel. Do not move up and down.

When teaching young students, after telling them to make their front stance, I reach around a doorway and pull a hidden lever. I make various machinery-like sound effects, then tell them I've just lowered the ceiling of the room until it is almost touching the tops of their heads. I further tell them the ceiling is paper-thin, and suspended above it is hot lava. (One of the benefits of owning your own dojo: the laws of physics are subject to your discretion.) They must move from one stance to the next without coming up and down at all.

You, too, can practice this skill, and no lava is required. Simply fix your gaze on a point opposite from you, on the wall or whatever it is you're looking at. As you do your C-step, take notice whether your eyes rise relative to that spot. Utilize this technique while practicing both forward and backward C-Steps.

If you prefer, you may use two papers' thickness!

Master Yutaka Yaguchi during the Instructor's Training Class
2006 ISKF Master Camp, Pennsylvania, USA

UKE AND TZUKI WITH C-STEP

Your next task is to add techniques to the C-Step. The techniques will be performed as you move.

Begin by stepping backward with jodan age uke. As your hips move backward, feel them rotating into a half-face position that is completed just as your rear foot comes to a stop. Execute your rising block as you move, just as you learned in the chapter on basics.[12] Its movement should end just as your hips and feet come to a stop. If your left leg is forward, your left arm should be blocking. Continue practicing stepping back, next with chudan ude uke, then with *gedan barai uke*.

When you perform your forward C-step, you can simultaneously punch using the same hand as the foot you're stepping with. Called *oi tzuki*, this is a handy technique for catching up to a retreating opponent, which is why it is sometimes called Chasing Punch as well as Lunge Punch or Stepping Punch.

The critical element in oi tzuki is to have the feeling that you are actually punching with your hips. Drive your hips toward your target and end with your hips in a straight-faced position. Your fist hits its imaginary target at the exact same moment that your front foot comes to a rest and your body locks into its proper forward stance. All must happen together, simultaneously.

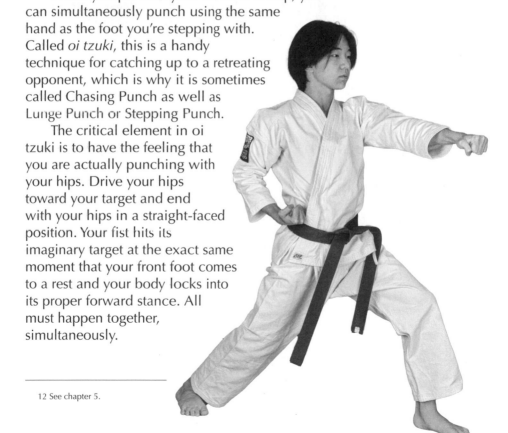

---

12 See chapter 5.

Oi Tzuki

Practice all blocks and all attacks moving forward and backward.

When you feel you are ready, you may add kicks to your C-step practice. Even though you are in front stance, a kick begins by bringing your knee up and pointing it to the target. Obviously, you can't keep your foot a paper's thickness from the floor if you are to do a kick. You can still do the C-step, however. Rather than tracing a C on the floor, your path will arc from the floor, where your foot was behind you, past your knee, then back down to the floor where your foot will land in front of you. Be sure to thrust your hips into the kick and not bob your head.

Bringing your legs together like this and bending your support leg so as to not rise in height stabilizes your body and provides the balance necessary for a strong kick. You can practice your backward C-step with kicking, too. Simply C-step back first, then lift your front knee, snap your kick out and back, and put your foot back down where it was. This is called *mayashi mae geri*. There should still be a feeling of thrusting your hips into the kick.

MAWATE

Turn or About-Face

The lessons available in your dojo may be infinite, but the size of the floor is not. Therefore, when Sensei has you perform your basic stepping drills, you'll eventually need to turn around and start heading in the opposite direction. As with every other activity that takes place on the dojo floor, this provides an opportunity for physical training and increased awareness.

When you reach the wall or end of the training area, become sensitive to the fact that your entire back is exposed. Imagine a hostile opponent trying to attack you on your exposed side. The turning method presented here offers a way to reduce the likelihood of being caught off-guard by such an attack.

Mawate is usually performed when, after performing a series of moving techniques, you find yourself facing a wall. If you've been practicing in front stance, bring your rear foot toward your front foot, keeping both knees bent so you stay low. That rear foot is about to become your front foot after you've turned. Rotate your torso 180° (do not switch feet, a common mistake) and drive aggressively in the new direction toward a new front stance.

The execution of the turn also gives you an opportunity to practice

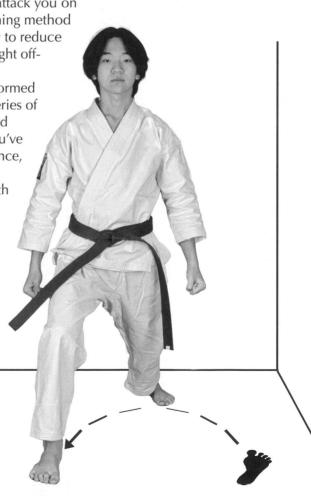

defending yourself. The most common defense made by beginners during mawate is a downward sweeping block, gedan barai uke, which is designed to defend the majority of your body against a deadly kick. Two other blocks are often used during mawate: if you had been training in mae geri, you should make a double downward block when you turn (as shown on page 71); if you had been training in back stance, then simply adjust your feet, rotate your posture, and perform a shuto uke in the opposite direction.

This practice should never be performed casually. To the contrary: when you hear the command, "Mawate!" you should imagine the sound of your sensei's voice to be the instant of an opponent's unexpected, malicious attack. Move at full speed and use a sharp *kiai* (a loud yell—see next chapter under *sambon kumite*). Do this *every* time you turn and you will become a challenging opponent indeed.

Chapter 9

Sparring

The very notion of *kumite,* or sparring, creates the greatest anxiety for many karatekas' personal relationships with karate. For some, the idea of having to get close enough with another individual to interact with their sweat and aggression is so repellent it ultimately drives them away from martial arts altogether. For others, aggression against another person, whether to satisfy personal bravado or to emulate Hollywood heroics, is the entire purpose of their martial art. Both groups misunderstand the larger concept and rob themselves of the extraordinary joys offered by Shotokan karate.

While you've learned basics, you've been working through a specific kinesiological system designed to maximize your focus and concentration of power. Practicing those fundamental movements against an opponent provides remarkable benefits in many aspects of your life. Think about it: despite what the Action and Adventure section of Netflix would have us believe, few of us have fists thrown toward our faces, ever, even once, thank goodness. When this first occurs in class, as it must, it may be traumatic to you, or may saturate your system with adrenaline. Both cause a loss of control. By the time you're ready to take your first Black-Belt exam, however, you'll have had thousands of fists in your face. The experience will no longer have any power to unsettle you. Knowing this, consider the many disheartening problems that occur in your life that pale in comparison to being punched in the face. How much better will you be able to handle those problems once being punched in the face is no big deal?

Understand sparring in its intended context. If you never need to defend yourself against an aggressor, but train thoroughly, you will have succeeded in your study of kumite. (I unapologetically explain my intent to my students: they will become well prepared for an event that will never happen.) To learn kumite is to learn *budo*, which means "to *stop* the fight," as Master Teruyuki Okazaki often said. Therefore, fighting cannot be the purpose of training in kumite. Rather, learning to understand oneself, and then, through compassion, learning to understand one's opponent enables more growth and achievement than any fight ever could.

THE VALUE OF STRUCTURE IN SPARRING

Many, many karate schools claim to offer "real" sparring. They do this by happily and profitably selling you head, face, chest, shin, forearm, foot, and hand protectors and sending you onto the training deck to face an opponent in a free-sparring match. Dressed like the Michelin Man with a white belt, you barely feel it when the opposing new student gives you his best shot. This renders impacts painless and, the argument goes, you can learn to execute techniques without fear of being hurt. But my experience has taught me to bet on a Black Belt trained in our unpadded method against an opposing Black Belt who came up through padded sparring any day.

There are problems with padding. First, there is reduced emphasis on learning to *not* be hit through body shifting and blocking. Students are given incentive to simply attack their opponents as often as possible; this means quantity over quality, pitter-patter over focused power. When I encounter a training partner who has learned to spar in this way, I usually find more openings than I can count. If he agrees to spar "my" way, unarmored, my friend's typical, flinching fear response—he feels so unprotected!—effectively reduces his competence as he tries to protect his many exposed areas. What would he do in a real-life encounter?

Self-Training

Ask a friend to be your target dummy. Have him or her stand a little more than an arm's length away from you while you're in shizen tai. Punching slowly, target jodan, meaning the mustache spot, with the first two knuckles of your perfectly-formed fist. Align your knuckles so they are precisely in that spot.

Practice moving one fist from draw-hand position to that jodan punch, then the other fist, repeatedly, at that same slow speed. Be careful. A martial artist must perfect self-control, which takes years. Never hit. Ever.

Then punch chudan, so your two knuckles would, another inch farther, insert themselves precisely into your friend's solar plexus. After several slow, targeted chudan punches, punch jodan again. Then move to gedan. Then jodan again.

You are isolating the invaluable practice of accuracy. Always move fluidly and slowly. In time, and as your sensei permits, you will learn to strike with incredible speed and power, and do so within a millimeter of your precise target. Do not increase your speed without the approval of your sensei. On your own time, however, you can improve your accuracy.

My second concern is that all of the body's vulnerable points are covered in the same amorphous foam, detracting from the variety of applications that can be deployed for various attack targets. This provides poor practice in the subtle variety of offensive techniques we are offered during kihon training.

My greatest worry is that wearing such gear may actually be *more* dangerous. The encouragement of less precise, less controlled attacks against thin foam armor is of grave concern. Additionally, my greatest anxiety about a strong roundhouse kick to the jaw is not a broken jaw. It's a broken neck. Padding the jaw doesn't change this. Learning the control necessary during unpadded sparring does.

When visitors watch White Belts sparring traditionally in Shotokan karate, they notice it doesn't look much like fighting at all. That's because it isn't like fighting. Not yet. For now, kumite is a drill intended to teach control of kihon —the basics already learned—while under the duress of a physical confrontation. To enable the karateka to focus on the quality of his techniques, the confrontation, for now, must be predictable and safe. My insurance company is very happy to hear that our objective is to *never* hit each other. (We hit foam shields, punching bags, *makiwara*, and other nonliving targets instead.)

Over time, we develop our techniques so they are incredibly fast, accurate, and powerful. That won't seem the case when watching most White Belts. But they, like you, are at a stage where those things are not of utmost importance. Proper technique is. During your first year of training, punches should land a good six inches from the targeted spot on your opponent. Ultimately you will be able to strike within millimeters of your target with speed and power—which means if you had wanted to hit your target, you easily could have. This kind of potent accuracy can only be achieved through the careful study of technique, which *sambon* and *gohon kumite* were developed to emphasize (see below). Speed and power can always be added. Try to understand that a fast, strong Black Belt who does not use good technique has many weaknesses.

AIMING

When they punch, strike, or even block in karate, many newer students are so concerned with the technique itself, they often neglect to focus on the *target* of the technique. Avoid the "Ready, Fire, Aim" syndrome. Know exactly where you're striking, every time, with surgical precision.

You'll hear the following terms for the entirety of your karate career. You would do well understand their specific meaning now.

REGIONS OF THE BODY

❖ **Jodan** includes the head and neck. When performing a jodan-level block, you want to envision defending your entire face, head, and neck. When attacking, however, you must practice great accuracy. When punching jodan, whether against a real or imagined opponent, target the area between the nose and upper lip—the mustache spot —with your first two knuckles. You may also be told to target the throat, eyes, or other soft targets, especially when using strikes. For obvious safety reasons, always proceed to these areas under your sensei's supervision.

❖ **Chudan** is your torso between your throat and belt. A proper chudan block, such as ude uke, ends its movement with the knuckles of the blocking hand level with the shoulder. If you position your hand there now, you will find the blocking surface of your wrist aligns itself perfectly to ward off an incoming attack to your solar plexus. The solar plexus is also the area you should target when you attack, again with your first two knuckles only. Eventually you will learn to target areas like the ribs, kidneys, and spine. Only do so under your sensei's direct guidance.

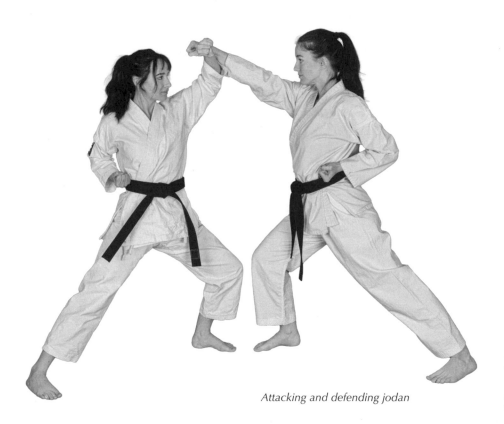

Attacking and defending jodan

❖ **Gedan** is everything below your belt. Areas you'll target when you are more advanced include your opponent's complex knee joint and the delicate metatarsal bones on the tops of his feet. For now, when attacking *gedan*, aim toward the groin. (Carefully!)

SAMBON KUMITE

Three-Step Sparring

Throughout your white, yellow, and orange belts and beyond, you will practice *sambon kumite*. If your dojo is of sufficient size, you may practice gohon kumite too, the only difference being that five steps are taken rather than three. Sambon or gohon kumite must be performed with strict adherence to its methodology and, of course, perfect etiquette. Review these steps several times so you are comfortable with the requirements of this drill when you are in the dojo. In this example, you will be the attacker first.

Always Begin with a Bow

Make musubi dachi and bow to your partner. When you rise from your bow, fix your gaze on your partner's eyes. Do not alter your gaze for the rest of the exercise.

You Attack to Jodan

1. Step back with your right leg, make a gedan barai with your left hand and a draw-hand to your hip with your right, and pronounce a sharp, loud yell known as a kiai. You may choose from three words for your kiai: "Ha!" "Sa!" or "To!" (pronounced "Tō").

2. Announce, "Oi tsuki jodan!" boldly, clearly, and confidently. (You've said, "I'd like to step in and punch your face, please.") Do nothing before your partner clearly replies, "Hai, jodan!" (Your partner has said, "I understand. Please do attack my face." See how extraordinary karate is? You've already had an experience most people never will.)

3. Commence your attack with an oi tzuki to jodan by C-stepping forward with your right foot and punching to the face with your right hand. Your partner will step back with his right foot and execute jodan age uke, also called rising block (as shown on page 78). Do this a total of three times or, in the case of gohon kumite, five times. Step rhythmically. You are to be predictable for your partner in this drill. Strategic manipulation of your opponent will come in future drills.

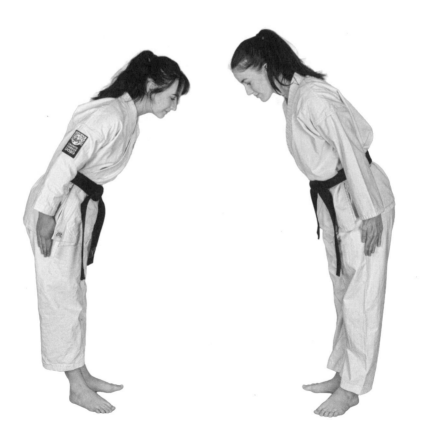

A note about safety: I'm writing this all out for you to study in comfort because, in the beginning, it is challenging to get it all right. But there is one mistake to avoid at all costs: you must *always* attack where you announce. Saying "Oi tzuki jodan!" and attacking chudan is a profound violation of etiquette and, obviously, dangerous. Be scrupulous when sparring. Keep your mind relaxed and clear.

4.   After blocking your last punch, keep your punching fist out for a moment. It serves as a block, making it more difficult for your partner to attack your face. He will therefore rotate his hips to straight-face and punch chudan toward your open stomach. *Do not block.* Simply hold your stance to allow your partner a chance to train in his offensive technique, as he has been for you.

Your Partner Attacks to Jodan

5.   After this, recover to shizen tai. Your partner will make gedan barai with a kiai, then announce, "Oi tzuki jodan!" Be sure you understand which hand you'll be attacked with, which foot you should step back with, and which hand you'll block with before you respond, "Hai, jodan!"

6.   Your partner will then attack toward your face with his right fist. You'll step back with your right leg and perform jodan age uke with your left hand. Step back and block two more times. While you are on defense, you must proceed according to the timing of your partner's attacks. Practice relaxing, focusing on your partner's eyes, and not moving before he does. This would create openings an advanced opponent could take advantage of. A relaxed state enables you to control your opponent, even though he is the one attacking.

7.   After the third attack, counterpunch with a gyaku tzuki to chudan.

Repeat the Process, This Time Attacking Chudan

8. Then, your partner recovers to shizen tai. Making gedan barai, you announce, "Oi tzuki chudan!" After your partner says, "Hai, chudan!" you commence an attack of three stepping punches to the stomach (shown below). This time, after your final oi tzuki, your partner counters to the face.

9. Recover to shizen tai and, after your partner announces "Oi tzuki chudan!" and you understand what you'll do, respond, "Hai, chudan!" Your partner will deliver three stepping punches to your stomach. Since his punching arm is somewhat in the way of his belly, counterpunch his face. Do so carefully of course, punching straight toward the spot between the upper lip and nose. Again, keeping a

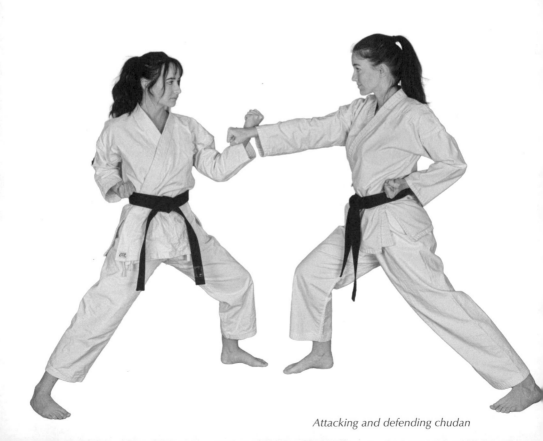

Attacking and defending chudan

good distance at first is prudent. You'll close that distance over time.

Change Sides, Do It All Again

10. As your partner recovers to shizen tai, switch your feet and make gedan barai uke with your right hand. Say, "Oi tzuki jodan!" and proceed with three stepping punches after your partner acknowledges his understanding of your intention. After your partner counterattacks, he will proceed to attack you three times. Block with three retreating rising blocks, then counterattack chudan.

> ### Self-Training
>
> *Invite a member in your family to a staring contest. That's something you may not have done for a very long time! Once you might have played this game to cause discomfort in your friend. This time, though, you're doing it to gain comfort and even relaxation during that gaze. Blink normally, and try for a minute, two minutes, or longer.*

11. Again your partner will recover to shizen tai while you make a right-handed gedan barai and announce, "Chudan oi tzuki!" As soon as he says, "Hai, chudan!" attack him with three stepping punches to his stomach. Then you'll counter his three attacks to your stomach with chudan ude uke and a single, final counter punch to jodan.

12. Change feet, and do it all again. Continue training for as long as you can until you hear your instructor's command to finish, *"Yame!"*

Always End with a Bow

Keeping your eyes on those of your partner, proper etiquette demands that you both recover to shizen tai. Then make musubi dachi; bow fully and respectfully, looking at your partner's feet. Rise, then make a shizen tai stance, returning your gaze to the eyes of your partner until you receive further instructions from your sensei.

Imagine yourself in a free-sparring situation against a competent Black Belt. There are virtually no rules other than those necessary for the safe, continued practice of karate. In that

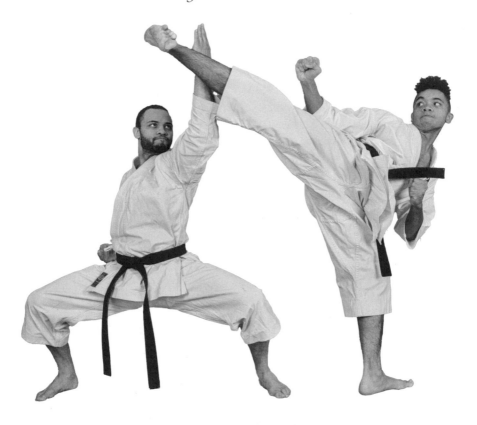

circumstance, you might be intimidated into a state of tension and poor self-control.

But imagine if I had years to prepare you for that match. Around that uncontrolled fight, I could begin to add restrictions— limitations that would allow for predictability and extreme focus on defined, individualized aspects of your sparring. Over years, we would piece those facets together, but not faster than you could develop comfort in each of them before adding it to the whole. Finally, you would face that freestyle match with a comfortable, relaxed awareness, confident you could control yourself *and* control your partner.

At one time or another, this seemed impossible to everyone now wearing a black belt. You'll get there.

Endeavor to excel.

Chapter 10

Kata: Heian Shodan

Self-Training

When you perform a kata, your steps trace a pattern on the floor. This pattern is known as an embusen, *and nearly every kata has a distinct one. The embusen are individualized further: they must be custom fit for the person performing the kata. Embusen are the snowflakes of Shotokan.*

You will be given a new kata to learn at least as often as you change belt colors in Shotokan karate. Now is the time to establish a place in your home where no one will mind if you use masking tape to create a pattern on the floor. Use the clarified embusen on page 87 as your guide. Mark the crosshatches first, each at a distance of twice your shoulders' width apart, which is the length of a good front stance. Then lay down the longer lines. (When you are more comfortable with the kata—when you have it "in your bones"—you might study the more complex embusen depicted on page 93.)

Practice your kata each night, even if you only do it a couple of times. If you keep to the cross marks, your muscle memory will become trained well in what a proper stance should look like. In class, you won't know any other way to stand, and your sensei will be impressed by how quickly you've learned your new kata.

Now you can begin your journey through the *kata*. These are forms composed of many movements to create mock battles against multiple opponents.

The kata are learned in order to provide development in specific skills at just the right time. Some kata are very old; they are considered cherished artifacts of history, each of which you must earn access to. For me, kata most embody the *art* of our martial art. There have been martial artists, brilliant by any measure, who *only* practiced kata. This is possible because they contain the catalog of our fighting tools. They are dances with deadly purpose.

During your time passing through the colored belts, you will learn all five of the *Heian* kata, a curriculum originally developed a century ago by Master Funakoshi's teacher Ankō Itosu, still practiced throughout the world. The Heians, originally called *Pinans* and considered to sit within the *shorin* category of kata, emphasize light, quick movements. Heian translates as "Peaceful Mind," a discovery made possible by their diligent practice even before you wear a black belt. *Heian Shodan*, or "Peaceful Mind First Step," will be taught to you after you have become acquainted with front stance, back stance, C-step, stepping punch, rising block, and knife-hand block.

The diagram pictured on page 89 is meant to be an aid as you as you review your kata at home. The pattern it follows is not the *embusen* (see sidebar) but is designed by the respected German karate teacher Albrecht Pflüger to enable a readable flow on a single page. It is quite accurate. Recalling what you've already learned in class, see if you can follow it along like a pictograph.

Then get up and do it.

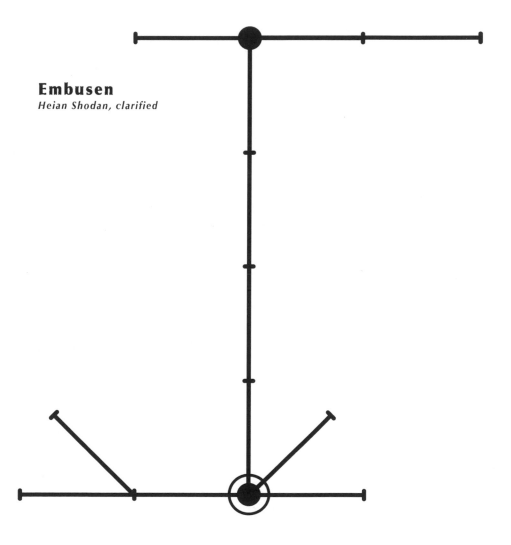

Embusen
Heian Shodan, clarified

After you've memorized the pattern of Heian Shodan, your chief concern during its practice should be the quality of the techniques that compose it. Look into your imaginary opponent's eyes rather than at the floor or some other place that doesn't hone your focus. Drive into stances that are consistent and correct. Rotate to straight-face when punching and half-face when blocking, and use a C-step when driving from one technique to the next. Keep your fists tight and your draw hand in its place. Strive for full relaxation. The more you relax, the more you will enjoy the snap of a powerful technique.

As any sincere martial artist would admit, that's a lot to absorb. But there is help to be found. A respectful request for help after class from a senpai will almost always meet with a positive reaction. Also, I encourage you to purchase Master Masatoshi Nakayama's definitive *Best Karate* series. You want these in your possession; we all refer to them often in our karate career, and you will, too. The Heian katas are contained in Volume 5.

Finally, practice often, incorporating these elements as much as possible. You need to get to the point where you're accustomed to the techniques you are called upon to perform in Heian Shodan, and at a level of quality that renders those techniques effective. At that point, your practice will benefit to the extent that you can imagine their use in a real situation. Really feeling the need for a strong block as you deploy it, yanking your wrist away during the escape, driving your punch in fully, and other attitudinal adjustments make the difference between those who go through the motions of their karate requirements and those who generate truly powerful focus.

FOCUS POINTS FOR HEIAN SHODAN[13]

❖ **#1: Gedan Barai**—The first movement of a kata is always vital, setting the tone for every subsequent movement. Experienced examiners can tell what to expect from the entire kata by watching a student's first technique. Make yours count. Collapse your structure nimbly, then drive

---

13 Use the numbers on the Pflüger diagram, page 89, when referencing these focus points.

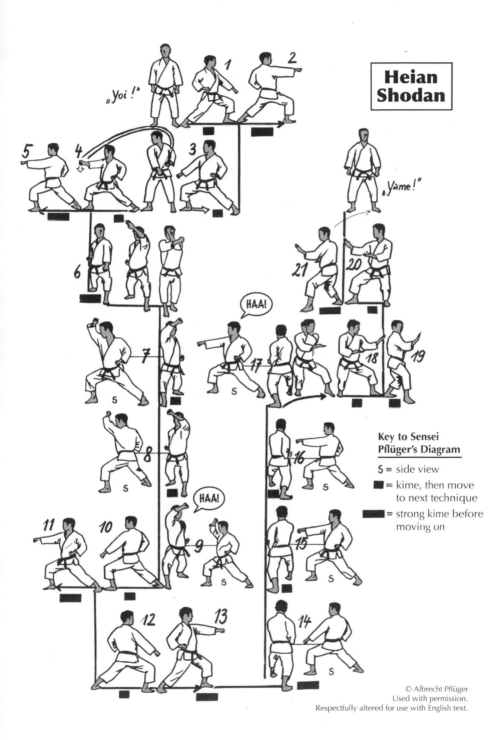

Heian Shodan

"yoi!"

"yame!"

HAA!

HAA!

Key to Sensei Pflüger's Diagram

S = side view

■ = kime, then move to next technique

▬ = strong kime before moving on

© Albrecht Pflüger
Used with permission.
Respectfully altered for use with English text.

your hips to the left explosively, imagining a powerful, incoming kick that needs deflecting.

❖ **#4: Escape and Kentsui**—After blocking his kick, your opponent has grabbed your right wrist with his left hand. By rotating your arm counter-clockwise against his thumb, you can escape your opponent's grasp. You should practice this with a partner. Heian Shodan further calls for you to escape vigorously, keeping your arm straight, and pushing it downward as you rotate. By coordinating this with a backward movement of the hips and the engagement of a strong *seika tanden*[14] (abdomen), a slender person can escape the grasp of a formidable man. Then, explode back, driving your hammer fist into your opponent's clavicle, disabling his ability to attack you further from that side.

❖ **#7–9: Jodan Age**—You might think you're blocking a three-armed opponent, but you are actually learning the practice of tai sabaki, or body shifting, as you aggressively drive into your opponent's position. After each rising block, open your hand and imagine grabbing the wrist of your opponent's arm, the one that just tried to punch you. The next block can be used as a break against that arm. After each block, you are to open your hand in a formal shuto, rather than a grasp. This will help you practice your self-control. If you can control your hand, you can easily grasp.

❖ **#10: Gedan Barai**—After the third rising block, you are required to bring your feet together, spin backward, and drive forward into a half-face stance, with feet hips' width apart. Why not simply block to your right instead? Be faithful: there are good reasons. With practice you will learn much from the required movement. Do not attempt to focus on the block. Focus instead on your body shifting forward, spinning, crossing your arms fully, and exploding to the right. Your block will become devastating.

---

14 More on this concept, as well as kime, is explored later in this book series.

❖ **#15–17: Oi Tzuki**—Similar to the three jodan blocks you performed earlier, these chudan punches are useful in learning to body-shift forward. Proper form is necessary to maximize power while maintaining control, however. Target your punch to an imaginary solar plexus correctly, and do not allow your momentum to throw you off balance.

❖ **#18–21: Shuto Uke/Uchi**—After implementing another challenging spin, you will deploy four precise knife-hand techniques. When you are ready, your instructor will reveal many interpretations of these four movements. They include blocks, grabs, strikes, breaks, and throws. Be sure to show a clear distinction between zenkutsu dachi and kokutsu dachi. Back stance should instantly feel dramatically different from front stance.

Self-Training

Practice Heian Shodan every day it is possible to do so, and perform as many repetitions of it as time allows. Your long-term goal is to rack up performances of the kata. Your one-hundredth Heian Shodan will feel much different than your one-thousandth, or your ten-thousandth. Some lessons are indescribable; there are those only available through achievement which, when it comes to kata, must be earned through repetition. At times, it is best to do so mindlessly, forgetting all of the many focus points there are to worry about. Get the quantity of practice under your obi (belt). You'll be rewarded with rich discoveries.

When you have experimented with the practical application of Heian Shodan's techniques, that is, its bunkai, you will have a strong basic understanding of its structure. The step pattern of the more detailed embusen seen on page 93 will become clear. From there, you will use the kata for many purposes. You will train with it regularly to seek technical excellence and new meaning from its tactics. You can practice variations of the kata, like mirror image (start with a downward block to the right, rather than to the left, and flow through a mirror of the kata's embusen), backward (starting with the last shuto uke, stepping backward through the embusen, and ending with the first gedan barai), and backward-mirror. You can perform the entire kata while pivoting on your left foot, enabling you to occupy only the space necessary to take a single step. At our school we practice another variation, generated from an insight provided by Master Hirokazu Kanazawa. He explained that katas contain forward-stepping defensive movements so as to not create the impression of militancy toward authorities at a time when Okinawa was occupied by Japan. Based on this speculation, my students perform the kata in what I call "inverse," where every block is accompanied by a step back, and all strikes are done while stepping forward. (Don't bother trying to end up back on your starting mark.) Kata can even be used as a pattern for practicing other techniques, so that after each strike or block, another technique is added, such as an in-place kick. It is possible to do a series of consistent movements and steps after each technique, like step-in/punch, step-back/block. One could even do an entire Heian Shodan after each move within Heian Shodan! Done correctly, it takes about twenty-one minutes and provides a great workout.

All of these practices generate a further awareness of Heian Shodan and the lessons it offers. Whenever performing any kata variation, however, be sure to "return to the beginning" by finishing your day's practice with a standard execution of the kata itself. Particularly in the case of Heian Shodan, you will find its clarity exhilarating, and your final kata will be the best of the day.

Embusen
Heian Shodan, detailed

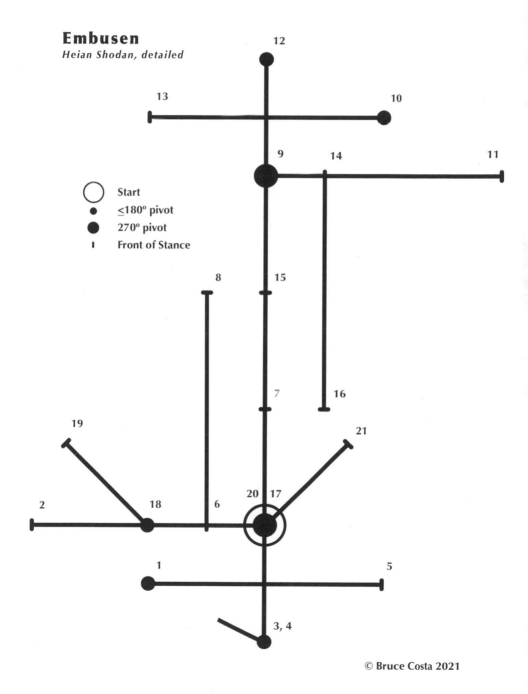

○ Start
● ≤180° pivot
⬤ 270° pivot
ı Front of Stance

© Bruce Costa 2021

Chapter 11

Encouragements

There are many elements to karate training left outside of a technical discussion of the art. Some of those elements can make a meaningful difference in your capacity to absorb and enjoy your training. Here are a few.

AWAKEN TO YOUR IMAGINARY OPPONENT

By practicing karate, you are training to be ready at any moment to defend yourself efficiently. You cannot defend yourself unless you recognize you are being threatened. The drudgery of daily tasks, poor nutrition, distractions, and other internal and external factors bring us in and out of alert awareness. Therefore, you must practice awareness. The dojo is an excellent awareness training center.

As you bow onto the dojo floor, wake up to all that is around you. Strive to maintain that consciousness until the time you bow off of the floor for the night. Your awareness should be at its utmost when you are practicing your techniques.

The next time you are standing in line waiting for a command in the dojo, set your eyes on a point on the wall opposite from you. Your practice is to focus on that one spot, thereby enabling all spots to come into your consciousness. You can visualize that spot as the eyes of an imaginary opponent: someone of your age, gender, weight, and height, with just a little bit more karate skill than you possess. Then, as you execute your techniques, you can make your experience more real as that person defends and counterattacks against you.

Awareness is a skill that all advanced karateka have worked hard to develop. It will benefit your karate tremendously if you do so, too.

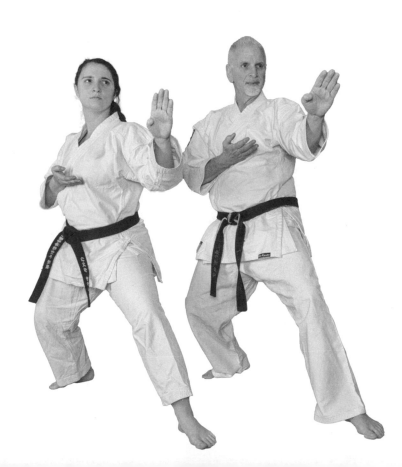

DEVELOP THE NOBILITY OF ZANSHIN

There will be many times you've completed your kata and Sensei callously leaves you struggling to maintain your final stance. Though your thighs and shoulder muscles may wail in complaint, hold your position diligently until Sensei says, *"Yame!"* indicating that you should return to shizen tai. This should be your practice at the end of any commanded drill, not just kata. It is within these moments that you will develop your capacity to hold out past the point you think you can—a skill karate practitioners are known for. In this context we call it the practice of *zanshin*, or "perfect finish." Zanshin also means "relaxed awareness." Its practice brings benefits to both mind and body that will be needed for the unusual and specific challenges karate will demand of them. When you hear the "Yame!" command, refocus on the imaginary opponent in front of you and recover to a perfect, strong shizen tai. It is in this moment, most of all, that you will seek perfection of character.

SMILE

There have been many, many times I *just did not want to* attend karate class! In those moments I had a dozen reasons not to go, ranging from kids to work to temptations of a less noble sort. During the years I lived an hour from my dojo, the commute often added to my list of "good" excuses to not train.

I had a dear friend, Daniel Rodman Walker, who passed away in 2001 from complications related to a lifelong struggle with kidney disease. He was a brilliant poet and a deep thinker. We had many tenacious, happy debates. Occasionally I posed what I thought was an unbeatable argument and sat back in my chair, content with my high-mindedness. Calmly, and only when I needed a good and appropriate drubbing, Danny would trump my point by saying, "You only think that way because you're healthy. Try being unhealthy and see if things change for you." Karate avoidance, I thought in times of reluctance, was one such application of my "healthy thinking" that Danny was unknowingly talking about. I would think of him tethered to a dialysis machine three times a week for six hours. He couldn't even attempt karate. What in the world did I have to whine about?

So I would play a game with myself. I would "see what happened." I wouldn't go to karate, I would simply go to the car and see what happened. As soon as I turned the ignition key, the book-on-tape would pick up where I'd left off and I was immediately involved. Why not drive and listen at the same time? My goal would then become to drive to a certain point on the journey to the dojo and see what happened when I got there. Invariably, when I'd reach that point, I was already too far along the way to reasonably turn back. Before I knew it, I was in my uniform and in class. Even at that point, there were times I felt less than enthused about being there. But I'd long since developed a mind-set that I'd fall over dead before walking off the dojo floor—even for reason of injury, exhaustion, or anything else—prior to the end of class. I knew once I was on the floor, I was in it until Sensei deigned to release me.

I can't recall for you how many times I felt this reluctance to attend karate. I can tell you, though, without any hesitation and with complete certainty, that *every single time* I manipulated myself into going to class, regardless of how much I didn't want to go, at the end of class I was glad I had attended it. Sometimes the desire to avoid karate was pronounced (doubting my competence as a karateka), sometimes the reasons seemed quite good (injury, money). Even at those times, when we closed our eyes for mokuso at the end of class, I'd feel the blood pumping through my limbs and the weight of my sweat-drenched gi and be overcome with gratitude. I'd be contemplating the incredible activity I had just participated in when suddenly I'd remember I hadn't wanted to come that night! What if I'd given in to my reluctance? I'd have missed the entire experience! At times the contrast between my initial resistance and my final accomplishment left me emotionally overwhelmed.

An old proverb says, "It is impossible to describe the taste of blowfish to one who has never eaten it." It should always be kept in mind that karate-do cannot be grasped through the eyes and ears alone; it must be experienced and comprehended through physical training.

Master Gichin Funakoshi
Karate-Do Nyūmon, 1943

Regardless of your physical condition when you begin your training and in spite of the hurdles you'll encounter during it, strive to keep in mind that you are, underneath it all, an athlete. We all are, by virtue of 300,000 years of evolution. Now you are invited to awaken muscles you've never used (even if you *are* athletic!) and see what they can do.

You get to do this. Many people can't. Be grateful.

Appendix 1

Written Exam

1) Brief Essay *(You may use more than the space provided.)*

What is the reason we bow?

_____

_____

_____

_____

_____

_____

2) Put the Dojo Kun in the order heard at the end of class:

_____   Endeavor to excel!
_____   Refrain from violent behavior!
_____   Be faithful!
_____   Seek perfection of character!
_____   Respect others!

3) Japanese Numbers:

one	_____	six	_____
two	_____	seven	_____
three	_____	eight	_____
four	_____	nine	_____
five	_____	ten	_____

4) Connect the Terms:

Kneel	Age Uke
Meditate	Dojo
Bow	Ude Uke
Finish	Zenkutsu Dachi
Senior	Gyaku Tzuki
Training studio	Kezami Tzuki
Front of training area	Senpai
Front stance	Rei
Back stance	Game
Jab punch	Oi Tzuki
Reverse punch	Shuto Uke
Stepping or lunge punch	Mocks
Downward block	Mae Geri
Forearm block	Seiza
Rising block	Shomen
Knife-hand block	Gedan Barai Uke
Front kick	Kokutsu Dachi

5) Fill in:

There are _____ steps in sambon kumite.

There are _____ steps in gohon kumite.

Our studio is called a _____.

The proper word for our teacher is _____.

The parts of the body are:

_____

_____

_____

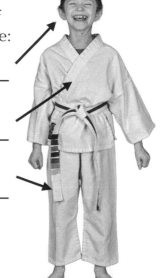

Appendix 2:
Practical Exam

In order to advance in karate rank, it is common for students to be reviewed in three specific, practical areas of training before receiving their yellow belts. These are kihon (basic techniques), kata (forms), and kumite (sparring).[15]

KIHON

You may be called upon to demonstrate proficiency in any of the following techniques, so it is best to practice them all thoroughly. Your acumen must be that of a Yellow Belt in each of these areas *before* you are awarded your yellow belt.

ZENKUTSU DACHI:	IN FRONT STANCE:
Oi Tzuki Jodan	Stepping punch to the face
Oi Tzuki Chudan	Stepping punch to the stomach
Jodan Age Uke	Rising block
Chudan Soto Ude Uke	Outward forearm block
Gedan Barai	Downward sweeping block
Mae Geri Keage Chudan	Front snapping kick to stomach
Mae Geri Keage Jodan	Front snapping kick to the face
KOKUTSU DACHI:	IN BACK STANCE:
Shuto Uke	Knife-hand block

---

15 These are the requirements of the International Shotokan Karate Federation as of this writing. Your organization's requirements may be different.

KATA

During your Yellow Belt exam you will be asked to perform Heian Shodan with proficiency. Key points to display are:

✓ Proper etiquette

✓ Good comportment

✓ Good spirit, involving the correct use of kiai

✓ Correct position and implementation of front stance

✓ Correct position and implementation of back stance

✓ Correct movement along the embusen (floor pattern)

✓ Correct use of front-face and half-face in strikes and blocks, respectively.

✓ Correct timing of the kata

✓ Zanshin (strong finish, relaxed awareness)

KUMITE

A proper demonstration of sambon kumite will require an understanding of the drill, good form under the stress of facing an opponent, and above all, excellent etiquette and sportsmanship.

Appendix 3

Ranking

Karate ranking for color-belts may differ slightly in various organizations. The International Shotokan Karate Federation's ranking proceeds as follows:

BELT COLOR	RANK
Yellow	8b Kyu
YOUR CURRENT GOAL ☞	8 Kyu
Orange	7b Kyu
	7 Kyu
Green	6b Kyu
	6 Kyu
Purple	5b Kyu
	5 Kyu
	4b Kyu
	4 Kyu
Brown	3b Kyu
	3 Kyu
	2b Kyu
	2 Kyu
	1b Kyu
	1 Kyu
Shodan, Nidan, Sandan, Yondan, etc.	

We are peculiar in our use of colored belts. Some martial arts schools don't use them at all. There is an argument to be made: should we not continually train simply for the benefit and joy of training? Indeed, no one gives you a different-colored weight belt at the gym, different-colored shoes at the dance studio, or different-colored goggles at the pool when you improve your level of performance. To this argument I would counter there is no activity I know of that is harder, and consequently more worthy of more intense study, than karate. These established checkpoints are a terrific help in guiding us along our path and keeping our training at the highest level. As a pianist's teacher suggests more challenging compositions to her students, we offer techniques, sparring conditions, and katas of increasing complexity. What's more, we all do better with deadlines before us. The warm accolades of your peers are welcome when you're handed your stiff, new, well-earned belt.

You'll notice there are two steps to every *kyu* (beginner or pre-black belt) level. If you take your first exam and receive a "b" in your ranking, it simply means the instructors noticed one thing or another that still needs practice. If you can become aware of this issue and address it, you will attain the level you're striving for at the next exam.

From this you are to take away the idea that there is no such thing as "failing" an exam. It's not a test, it's an exam, as in exam*ination*—a look—by people more experienced than you, at where you are right now. For this reason, you should take advantage of every exam opportunity you can.

And you shouldn't concern yourself with the color of your belt. With regard to both advancement and exams (whether they be kyu, dan, or instructor exams), remember this most of all:

❖ If you take your exam and find you have reached your desired level, you will come back to classes and train in karate.

❖ If you take your exam and find you have *not* reached your desired level, you will come back to classes and train in karate.

The next book in this series is appropriate for those who have achieved a yellow belt and a rank of 8b kyu or 8 kyu. In it, and in your own study of karate, you will be introduced to a complex, exciting, and beautiful kata known as Heian Nidan. It will reveal several new and very effective techniques, such as outward forearm block (*uchi uke*), side snap kick (*yoko geri keage*), and reverse half face (*gyaku hanmi dachi*). You will become more proficient with the kicks, punches, and strikes you've already learned and also in their application to sparring.

It is an exciting time for you. Keep training.

Appendix 4

Your Uniform

CHOOSING A GI

There are many uniforms available for purchase. The traditional "Japanese" gi is made all over the world. As mentioned earlier, I encourage you to support your dojo by buying from what is available there. There may be three or more qualities offered:

❖ A **light-weight** gi would be your most economical choice and may be the only choice for a young child. It will be constructed of a five- to six-ounce cotton/polyester blend. As a result it won't absorb much perspiration and can cling uncomfortably to your skin if you sweat heavily. The pants will have an elastic waistband. A light-weight gi is plenty durable and makes a fine choice for a first uniform.

❖ A **medium-weight** uniform will be made from a nine- or ten-ounce fabric that can be 100-percent cotton but is more commonly a cotton/polyester blend. It has more absorption capacity than a light-weight gi and is often marginally more expensive.

❖ A **heavy-weight** gi is the only gi I will wear. I don't know of a Black Belt who wears anything else. Heavy-weight gis are costlier, but their capacity to absorb sweat is unmatched. They can be made of a cotton-poly blend or 100-percent cotton. In the latter case, different manufacturers treat their cotton differently. Some uniforms feel like you're wearing an artist's canvas, while others are brushed and feel exquisite. In my experience, cost is not related to comfort or performance. I have a $130 gi that I greatly prefer to my $300 gi. A 100-percent-cotton gi is prone to wrinkling, but those of us who are iron-averse are willing to put up with a few wrinkles for this level of quality. I think any Black Belt would have to admit the foremost reason he wears a heavy-weight gi is for the nice snapping sound it makes when doing a good karate technique!

CARING FOR YOUR GI

Hem it.

Consider yourself lucky if you find a gi that fits you without being hemmed. Most of us need to do some stitching—no easy task when you have a heavy-weight gi! Be sure to feed it slowly through your sewing machine. I've bent many needles.

Many people like to wear their uniforms at the same length as they would their business suits. I have a couple of uniforms at this length that I keep white and pressed for self-defense presentations to business groups or motivational lectures to schools. But I like a shortened uniform for training. Some higher-end gi manufacturers even sell variations that arrive already shortened. The rule for hemming is that the pants can be no shorter than half way up your calf and the jacket no shorter than half way up your forearm.

Patch it.

If your dojo is affiliated with a larger organization, wear its patch, along with that of the dojo itself. I encourage you to attach these immediately and professionally. Wear them proudly. Consider doing so a part of the Zen of Giving Service.

There are, however, schools that go overboard in adorning their uniforms with huge logos on the back and all manner of bangles and frippery from shoulder to ankle. This is unnecessary, and contrary to the spirit of simplicity that surrounds our practice. The children in my dojo receive award patches for our long-range goal program and for getting good grades on their report cards, but they are confined to a small area of the shoulder and arranged in an unobtrusive fashion. Our school is about learning, not gilding.

Wash it.

You can wash your uniform as you would any white garment. I use only a moderate amount of bleach and prefer spot treatments so as to not blanch the patches. If you're training as often as you should, you'll find you need more than one gi just to become less enslaved to the washing machine. I have six.

CARING FOR YOUR BELT

I am told that not too long ago, in Japan, there were no such things as colored karate belts, or *obi*. They all were made white. But there was a tradition that the belt was special. It was not to be laid about, or washed, ever. Obviously, the more one trained, the dirtier his belt would get. If you came upon someone wearing a *black* belt, you knew he had been at it for some time.

We keep that tradition. Take good care of your obi. Never let it lay on the ground. When you've become a Yellow Belt, display your white belt nicely. When you find yourself struggling with the challenges that come with your yellow belt, that display can encourage you as a reminder of earlier accomplishments. Those were hard, too. Be faithful. You'll get through it.

When I put on my obi, I try to remember the special possession it is, the years it has seen, and the journey I took before I was entitled to it. It helps me remember that I may be a little bit ahead of you, but I'm on the same path you are. I hope you'll enjoy tying your belt as much as I do mine.

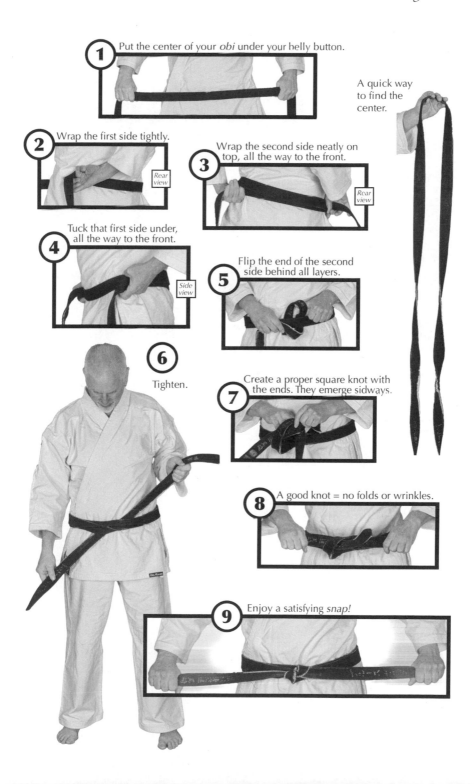

1 Put the center of your *obi* under your belly button.

A quick way to find the center.

2 Wrap the first side tightly.

Rear view

3 Wrap the second side neatly on top, all the way to the front.

Rear view

4 Tuck that first side under, all the way to the front.

Side view

5 Flip the end of the second side behind all layers.

6 Tighten.

7 Create a proper square knot with the ends. They emerge sidways.

8 A good knot = no folds or wrinkles.

9 Enjoy a satisfying *snap!*

Homage: The Mountain

The food was in front of the kids. Lynn felt a moment of hope: she needed only to put the leftovers away and she might actually be able to eat her dinner while it was still hot.

Her cell phone rang. Terry's face, twisted into a goofy expression, popped up on the screen. She smiled at it despite his timing. She loved him, but he was late getting home from work as it was, and if this was one of his philosophical rants…

"Yes…" Her voice was expectant, impatient, and sarcastic all at once.

"I know I'm late and there's gonna be a cold dinner waiting for me…" Terry's voice was excited, unsettled.

Through the phone, Lynn heard Terry rapidly shift into park and jangle his keys as he killed the ignition. "Sounds like you've got stuff going on," she said. "I guess I'll wrap up your dinner."

"I just need to stop into the dojo for a second. Go ahead and eat."

When she heard the bedroom door open over two hours later, Lynn kept her nose firmly planted in her book. "That was some second," she said in the same tone of voice she'd used earlier. "Your dinner's on the bottom fridge shelf. Red Tupperware."

There was no answer. No guilt-drenched apology, either—which normally was a Terry tradition after a multi-hour dojo-related disappearance. A moment went by. Then another. Something was different. Lynn looked up.

Terry was standing over his dresser where he normally engaged in the pre-undressing ritual of emptying his pockets. But he was just standing there, utterly lost in thought, as if he had forgotten what it was he was supposed to do. Then she noticed something else: Terry's suit pants were dirty, and his normally meticulous Oxfords were scuffed. His father had given him those shoes. That he would be careless in them seemed inconceivable. What Lynn cared about, though, were her taupe carpets. She had long since housebroken her husband to leave his shoes, even unscuffed ones, by the back door.

She pushed aside the death threats taking shape in her mind and allowed her voice to turn compassionate. "Honey, what happened?"

No sign of life. "Honey?"

"Huh? Oh! Sorry. I was just…thinking."

The threats pushed their way back. "No!" Lynn's eyes grew wide. "Really? I'd never have known! I thought that was conversation! You want to tell me what happened, and *why* I shouldn't kill you for tracking dirt across the carpet?"

"Oh crap!"

After removing his shoes and swearing a solemn oath to steam clean, Terry washed up. As he put on his pajamas he grew quiet again, and Lynn found the silence a distraction from her reading. He got into bed and reached neither for the book he was nearly finished reading nor for her. Lynn watched as his eyes found something of interest very far away.

That was it. She elbowed him. Hard.

"OWWW! Jeez! What was that for?"

"If you don't tell me what happened I'm gonna do it again!"

Terry smiled. "Look, this whole karate thing…" and, rubbing his sore upper arm, he added, "…which you'd be *very* good at, by the way…it's been getting to me. I had to talk to Sensei about it.

"But when I got to the dojo, Sensei wasn't there. No one knew where he was. As I was leaving, one of the instructors stuck her head out from the office and said when no one knows where Sensei is, he's usually at the state park.

"It was on the way home, so it was easy to stop and see if his car was there. I found it…at the Lenape Trailhead."

"The Lenape Trail is the one that goes all the way up the mountain," Lynn said.

"Yeah. Tell me about it."

"Wait, you're telling me you hiked that trail? In your office clothes?"

"I figured, look, the guy's not a spring chicken. I jogged up the trail, figuring I wouldn't have to go far to catch him. When I got halfway up the mountain the jog became a climb. A pretty intense climb, actually. I emerged at the top to one of the most beautiful sunsets I'd ever seen. Sensei was just sitting on one of the rocks, facing the sunset."

Terry smiled. "I actually thought about seeing if I could sneak up on him! But he turned 'round and said, 'Mr. Farrell! What a coincidence!' I was like, 'Damn, this guy's good!'"

"I said, 'Not such a coincidence, Sensei. I was hoping to ask you a question.' I felt like I should have bowed to him, but I felt funny enough as it was, hiking a hard trail in my work clothes, so I didn't.

"He said, 'Must be an important question to chase me up here for it. I sure hope I brought an answer.'

"I said, 'Sensei, there are days when I feel like I'm just lousy at karate. I make so many mistakes! I'm not used to that. I'm thinking maybe I'm just not cut out for it.' And he said, 'Yeah.'"

"He said, 'yeah?'"

"Yeah."

"Ouch."

"Oh, it gets worse," Terry said without looking up. "He said, 'So is there anything else?' He never stopped looking at the horizon. I asked if he thought I had any chance at all, if he thought I could get any good at it, if I did stick with it."

"Honey, you've been thinking of quitting?" Lynn felt shocked. Ever since she met him fresh out of the military, no matter how tough the challenge, she'd never known Terry to give up at anything. "You've done so much. I just figured karate was another thing you'd check off."

"Yeah, I've been going back and forth in my head about it. I mean, I've got an amazing life, you know? I do well in my career, I have a great family. Why bang my head against the wall? But it does feel amazing when I get it right, and I must say, it drives me nuts to think I might not keep going. I should be able to plan this out and pull it off. In the Navy I learned to set goals, work hard, and achieve them. I learned that the clearer the picture, the more likely I'd achieve the goal. My black belt in karate should be like that, right? I just didn't realize even the beginning steps would be this hard. I needed some clarity on it. I figured, who better to ask than my teacher? So then he said, 'Tell me what you really want to ask me,' and I said, 'I was wondering how long you thought it might take for me to get my black belt.'

"'Ah,' he said, 'the very thing inquiring White Belts want to know.'

"So what did he say?"

"He asked me if I had ten bucks."

"Huh?"

"That's what *I* said. But he said, 'Ten bucks. Go back to the dojo, tell them I said you could buy one, right now.' Freaked me out."

"I would think so," Lynn said.

"Then he said, 'There's a catch.' He said I'd have to start taking Black Belt classes right away."

"You'd get killed!"

"Yeah, that's what I said. He agreed. I told him I want to train for it, that I want to do what it took for everyone else to get their black belts. He said, 'I'm sure you do.' I would have thought he was mocking me, but he was, like, really nice about it. It was weird. So I asked him how long it would take me to get it if I trained twice a week. He said, 'Five years.'"

Lynn said, "That's it? Just a straight answer? Cool! So why didn't you just come home? You got your answer, free of philosophical mumbo-jumbo."

"Oh, don't worry," Terry smiled. "That's coming. I asked him how long it would take if I trained three times every week. He said, 'Ten years.'

"I said, 'No, Sensei, I mean what if I train 50 percent more?'

"He said, 'Yes, I understood. Ten years.'

"'Okay...what if I train every day?'"

"Lemme guess," Lynn said. "Fifteen years?"

"You got it. Honestly, after that climb I was feeling a little jerked around."

"I'll bet," Lynn said. "Honey, have you thought about other karate schools?"

Terry was smiling. "Sure I have. But I want a great teacher, and I'm telling you, this guy is one. He finally let me off the hook. He said, 'Mr. Farrell (he always calls me that!), on your hike up here to see me, did you fall off the trail? During the hundreds of steps, wearing those slippery shoes, did you fall off, even once?'

"I hadn't, of course. I was pretty focused.

"He said, 'It's a tough trail. Did you consider turning back?'

"'After I'd hiked a while and didn't see you, sure,' I said.

"He said, 'And for your persistence you got this beautiful sunset.'

"And this brain-melt, I thought.

"He said, 'So you didn't fall. Where were your eyes looking as you hiked?'

"'At the trail,' I said. I didn't want to walk off a cliff. I figured, with how late I was already, and now on this cockamamie expedition, dying would really get me in trouble back home.

"He asked me if I believed I'd make it to the summit if I kept hiking. I told him, sure, if I kept going I figured I'd make it there eventually. Then he smiled at me."

"This guy's weird," Lynn said.

"No doubt. Then he said, 'Of course, if you kept your eyes on the top of the mountain, you could have better calculated the exact moment of your arrival. Mr. Farrell, have you memorized the promises we make at the end of each class yet?'

"I had to say, 'No, Sensei, in fact I can only repeat the English version of the Dojo Kun right now.'

"He said, 'That's fine. Do you remember the second sentence we say?'

"I did remember. I said, 'Be Faithful.'

"'Mr. Farrell,' he said, 'you knew if you did not abandon the trail, and simply kept moving forward, you'd come to the top of the mountain. You could not see the top, but you got there by focusing on the immediate. Your faith kept you aware of the goal, but you achieved it by living in the present moment—which is really the only moment you possess. Therefore, to some extent, you must abandon your goal in order to achieve it.'

"I noticed him looking at my face; I must have looked confused. He looked compassionate. He said, 'Do you remember the part of the trail where you *can* see the top of the mountain?'

"'Yeah,' I said, 'it's the section along the cliff. There's nowhere for trees to grow, so it's clear and you have a view of the top. It's a great view. You have to stop walking, though.'

"'Why?'

"'Because you'll fall off and die!' I said. 'You have to pay attention to where you are!'

"'Just like karate,' he said. 'The extent to which you concern yourself about your black belt is the extent to which you delay its arrival. But if you practice diligence, and let meditation bring you to the present moment, you'll have your black belt before you know it.'

"We sat quietly together for a while. Then we walked down the mountain together, again mostly in silence. I needed to think, and it was as if Sensei perceived and respected that.

"And now, sitting here with you, the karate path seems foggier than ever, and yet...I can't believe I'm gonna say this about something I don't understand, but..." Terry trailed off.

"But what?"

"I don't know if my subconscious figured something out that I can't describe or if it's just out of respect for Sensei, but I feel like I really want to keep doing this. Like, more than ever. I swear to God I could go train right now."

"Wow. So, is that the end of the story?"

"Almost. I asked him why it would take so *much* longer to get my black belt—five extra years for training three times a week, and so forth.

"He said, 'You'd need time for your bruises to heal.'"

Postscript

A PERSONAL NOTE

As of this writing, I've been training in karate for over four decades. It remains an exhilarating activity for me. Compared to a more youthful time, with too many memories of being bullied, karate now brings a sense of control and serenity. As a result, facing another person in sparring is far from the source of stress and tension it once was. Indeed, it is among the most thrilling aspects of my martial art—and not because of the violence of it. Relationships progress in such confrontations. Strangers become friends, friends become confidantes. Invariably, I come away from a karate encounter closer to my training partner than I was when I began it.

I am proud to be able to tell you that my only confrontational use of karate in my entire life has been in such matches.

I take pains to express this pleasure to each of my students at the beginning of their time with me. I tell them a good martial artist understands the true lesson of tai sabaki—of simply not being in the path of a blow. This can involve body shifting in the moment of an attack or walking to school along a different route than the one where thugs linger.

There is another reason I avoid fights that is more important to me than my personal safety. As any competent karateka will tell you, the self-control Shotokan brings also enables an extraordinary focus of power. These techniques can crush bones. By any reasonable interpretation, this is not cool. It's destructive. Here is the way I explain this to classes of young children:

> *What would I try to do if a big, scary man tried to hurt me? First, I'd talk to him. My mouth is more agile than my hands, so my words will always express myself better than my fists will. Only by talking will I discover the truth: Maybe he's upset about something. Maybe I can help him. Because, you see, if I hit him, it wouldn't be like it is on TV. After I hit him, his eye wouldn't work, any more, ever. He would have to go to the hospital. His friends would visit him there and feel sad. His mom would cry. If you cover one eye with your hand, you'll see what the world would look like for him when he came out of the hospital. It would look like that every day, forever.*

I don't want to do that to anyone. I want to be nice. I want to lead a peaceful, helpful life. I want that for you, too. Refrain from violent behavior. Use your karate to learn how to learn. With it, you can unveil the best person that already lies within you.

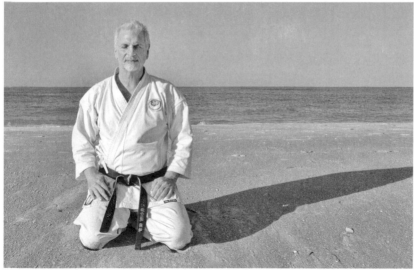

Sensei Rick Hotton's Winter Keiko, Sarasota, Florida.

Glossary

STANCES (DACHI)

Natural stance	Shizen Tai
Front stance	Zenkutsu Dachi
Back stance	Kokutsu Dachi

BLOCKING (UKE)

Downward block	Gedan Barai Uke
Forearm block	Ude Uke
Rising block	Age Uke
Knife hand block	Shuto Uke

PUNCHING (TZUKI)

Jab punch	Kezami Tzuki
Reverse punch	Gyaku Tzuki
Stepping or lunge punch	Oi Tzuki

STRIKING (UCHI)

Knife hand strike	Shuto Uchi
Hammer fist strike	Kentsui

KICKING (GERI)

Front kick	Mae Geri
Front leg kick	Mayashi Mae Geri

SPARRING (KUMITE)

Five-attack sparring	Gohon Kumite
Three-attack sparring	Sambon Kumite

VARIOUS NOMENCLATURE

Upper level (head)	Jodan
Middle level (torso)	Chudan
Lower level (groin)	Gedan
Ready	Yoi
Bow	Rei
Begin	Hajime
Finish	Yame
Kneel	Seiza
Meditate	Mokuso
Shout	Kiai
Body center, abdomen	Seika Tanden
Senior	Senpai
Junior	Kohai
Ready position	Kamae Te
Training studio	Dojo
Front of training area	Shomen

COUNTING

One	Ichi
Two	Ni
Three	San
Four	Shi
Five	Go
Six	Roku
Seven	Sichi
Eight	Hachi
Nine	Ku
Ten	Ju

Pronunciation Guide

ENUNCIATION

Japanese enunciation may sound so unfamiliar as to be confusing to you. Becoming aware of a couple of key differences in our linguistics, however, will help you follow along. For illustration, here are the numbers one through ten:

ichi	ni	san	shi	go
roku	sichi	hachi	ku	ju

It is common to truncate vowels at the end of multi-syllabic words. Accordingly, *"ni"* (the number two) is pronounced "nee," but *"roku"* (the number six) is pronounced "rōke." There is also no syllabic emphasis, unlike Latin-based languages. Therefore, when speaking a Japanese word, give all syllables the same emphasis.

JAPANESE	ENGLISH	PRONUNCIATION
Age Uke	Rising Block	ah-gay oo-kay
Choku Tzuki	Straight Punch	chō-koo tsoo-kee
Chudan	Middle Level (Torso)	choo-dahn
Dachi	Stance	dah-chee
Dojo	Training Studio	dō-jō
Dojo Kun	Studio Promise	dō-jō koon
Embusen	Kata Floor Pattern	em-byoo-sen
Gedan	Lower Level (Groin)	gay-dahn
Gedan Barai	Downward Block	gay-dahn bah-raī
Geri	Kick	gay-ree
Gi	Karate Uniform	gee
Gohon Kumite	Five-Attack Sparring	gō-hōn koo-mee-tay
Gyaku Tzuki	Reverse Punch	gyah-koo tsoo-kee
Hai	Yes	haī
Hajime	Begin	hah-jee-may

JAPANESE	ENGLISH	PRONUNCIATION
Heiko Dachi	Parallel Stance	hay-kō dah-chee
Jodan	Upper Level (Head)	jō-dahn
Kamae Te	Ready Position	kah-maī tay
Karateka	Student of Karate	kah-rah-tay-kah
Kata	Choreographed Forms	kah-tah
Kentsui	Hammer Fist Strike	kehn-tsoo-ee
Kezami Tzuki	Jab Punch	kay-zah-mee tsoo-key
Kiai	Shout	kee-aī
Kihon	Basic Techniques	kee-hōn
Kohai	Junior	kō-haī
Kokutsu Dachi	Back Stance	kō-koo-tsoo dah-chee
Kumite	Sparring	koo-mee-tay
Mae Geri Keage	Front Snap Kick	mah-yay gay-ree kay-ah-gay
Makiwara	Punching Post	mah-key-wah-rah
Mayashi Mae Geri	Front Leg Kick	mah-yah-shee mah-yay gay-ree
Mokuso	Meditate	moh-koo-sō
Musubi Dachi	Knot Stance	moo-soo-bee dah-chee
Obi	Belt	ō-bee
Oi Tzuki	Stepping Punch	oy-tsoo-kee
Rei	Bow	ray
Sambon Kumite	Three-Attack Sparring	sahm-bōn koo-mee-tay
Seika Tanden	Abdomen	say-kah tahn-dehn
Seiza	Kneel	say-zah
Senpai	Senior	sehn-paī
Sensei	Instructor	sehn-say
Shizen Tai	Natural Stance	shee-zehn taī
Shomen	Front Of Training Area	shō-men
Shuto Uchi	Knife Hand Strike	shoo-tō oo-chee
Shuto Uke	Knife Hand Block	shoo-tō oo-kay

JAPANESE	**ENGLISH**	**PRONUNCIATION**
Tai Sabaki	Body Shifting	taī sah-bah-kee
Tzuki	Punching	tsoo-kee
Uchi	Strike	oo-chee
Ude Uke	Forearm Block	oo-day oo-kay
Uke	Block	oo-kay
Yame	Finish	yah-may
Yoi	Ready	yoy
Zanshin	Relaxed Awareness	zahn-shin
Zenkutsu Dachi	Front Stance	zehn-koo-tsoo dah-chee

Student Journal

With all the encouragement I can muster, I offer you space to briefly journal after your early training experiences. All of us with black belts worn white wish we had our early struggles better captured. We'd happily rediscover escaped memories and moments of discovery. We'd increase our compassion with our students. But first, we'd smile, and even laugh. Should you find this craft as engaging as we have, you'll be glad this time is documented. Use these pages to capture your thoughts. Use video to capture your performance. You'll have eyes that look at yourself differently one day.

Class #_____ Day _____ Date ____/____/____

_____

_____

_____

_____

_____

Class #_____ Day _____ Date ____/____/____

_____

_____

_____

_____

_____

Class #_____ Day _____ Date ____/____/____

_____

_____

_____

_____

_____

Class #_____ Day _____ Date ____/____/____

_____

_____

_____

_____

_____

Class #_____ Day _____ Date ____/____/____

_____

_____

_____

_____

_____

Class #_____ Day _____ Date ____/____/____

_____

_____

_____

_____

_____

Class #_____ Day _____ Date ____/____/____

_____

_____

_____

_____

_____

Class #_____ Day _____ Date ____/____/____

_____

_____

_____

_____

_____

Class #_____ Day _____ Date ___/___/___

_____

_____

_____

_____

_____

Class #_____ Day _____ Date ___/___/___

_____

_____

_____

_____

_____

Class #_____ Day _____ Date ___/___/___

_____

_____

_____

_____

Class #_____ Day _____ Date ____/____/____

_____

_____

_____

_____

_____

Class #_____ Day _____ Date ____/____/____

_____

_____

_____

_____

_____

Class #_____ Day _____ Date ____/____/____

_____

_____

_____

_____

_____

Class #_____ Day _____ Date ____/____/____

_____

_____

_____

_____

_____

Class #_____ Day _____ Date ____/____/____

_____

_____

_____

_____

_____

Class #_____ Day _____ Date ____/____/____

_____

_____

_____

_____

_____

Class #_____ Day _____ Date ____/____/____

_____

_____

_____

_____

_____

Class #_____ Day _____ Date ____/____/____

_____

_____

_____

_____

_____

Class #_____ Day _____ Date ____/____/____

_____

_____

_____

_____

_____

Class #_____ Day _____ Date ____/____/____

_____

_____

_____

_____

_____

Class #_____ Day _____ Date ____/____/____

_____

_____

_____

_____

_____

Class #_____ Day _____ Date ____/____/____

_____

_____

_____

_____

_____

Class #_____ Day _____ Date ____/____/____

_____

_____

_____

_____

_____

Class #_____ Day _____ Date ____/____/____

_____

_____

_____

_____

_____

Class #_____ Day _____ Date ____/____/____

_____

_____

_____

_____

_____

Class #_____ Day _____ Date ____/____/____

_____

_____

_____

_____

_____

Class #_____ Day _____ Date ____/____/____

_____

_____

_____

_____

_____

Class #_____ Day _____ Date ____/____/____

_____

_____

_____

_____

_____

ABOUT THE AUTHOR

Bruce Costa has presented and taught throughout North America and Western Europe, and has been privileged to train with some of the finest karate instructors and practitioners in the world for over four decades. He is the father of three happy adults, all of whom are Shotokan Black Belts. You can read more at BruceCosta.com.

In 2002 Sensei Costa established Granite Forest Dojo. Today its membership includes focused preschoolers, spirited tournament champions, hearty senior citizens, superb instructors, and many high-achieving Black Belts. The facility was hand-made by these people over the course of two years. Granite Forest Sangha is hosted there, offering mindfulness meditation in the tradition of Thich Nhat Hanh, with whom Mr. Costa has practiced since 2007. Along with its faculty, students, and their families, Granite Forest Dojo helped The Christopher Court Foundation raise hundreds of thousands of dollars for pediatric tumor research in honor of Sensei Costa's young student. You can visit this welcoming dojo personally in Bucks County, Pennsylvania, or virtually at GraniteForestDojo.org.

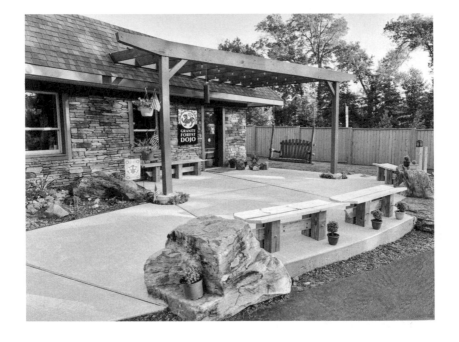

BOOKS FROM YMAA

VIDEOS FROM YMAA

ADVANCED PRACTICAL CHIN NA IN-DEPTH
ANALYSIS OF SHAOLIN CHIN NA
ATTACK THE ATTACK
BAGUA FOR BEGINNERS 1
BAGUA FOR BEGINNERS 2
BAGUAZHANG: EMEI BAGUAZHANG
BEGINNER QIGONG FOR WOMEN 1
BEGINNER QIGONG FOR WOMEN 2
BEGINNER TAI CHI FOR HEALTH
CHEN STYLE TAIJIQUAN
CHEN TAI CHI CANNON FIST
CHEN TAI CHI FIRST FORM
CHEN TAI CHI FOR BEGINNERS
CHIN NA IN-DEPTH COURSES 1—4
CHIN NA IN-DEPTH COURSES 5—8
CHIN NA IN-DEPTH COURSES 9—12
FACING VIOLENCE: 7 THINGS A MARTIAL ARTIST MUST KNOW
FIVE ANIMAL SPORTS
FIVE ELEMENTS ENERGY BALANCE
INFIGHTING
INTRODUCTION TO QI GONG FOR BEGINNERS
JOINT LOCKS
KNIFE DEFENSE: TRADITIONAL TECHNIQUES AGAINST A DAGGER
KUNG FU BODY CONDITIONING 1
KUNG FU BODY CONDITIONING 2
KUNG FU FOR KIDS
KUNG FU FOR TEENS
LOGIC OF VIOLENCE
MERIDIAN QIGONG
NEIGONG FOR MARTIAL ARTS
NORTHERN SHAOLIN SWORD : SAN CAI JIAN, KUN WU JIAN,
    QI MEN JIAN
QI GONG 30-DAY CHALLENGE
QI GONG FOR ANXIETY
QI GONG FOR ARMS, WRISTS, AND HANDS
QIGONG FOR BEGINNERS: FRAGRANCE
QI GONG FOR BETTER BALANCE
QI GONG FOR BETTER BREATHING
QI GONG FOR CANCER
QI GONG FOR DEPRESSION
QI GONG FOR ENERGY AND VITALITY
QI GONG FOR HEADACHES
QI GONG FOR HEALING
QI GONG FOR THE HEALTHY HEART
QI GONG FOR HEALTHY JOINTS
QI GONG FOR HIGH BLOOD PRESSURE
QIGONG FOR LONGEVITY
QI GONG FOR STRONG BONES
QI GONG FOR THE UPPER BACK AND NECK
QIGONG FOR WOMEN
QIGONG FOR WOMEN WITH DAISY LEE
QIGONG FLOW FOR STRESS & ANXIETY RELIEF
QIGONG MASSAGE
QIGONG MINDFULNESS IN MOTION
QI GONG—THE SEATED WORKOUT
QIGONG: 15 MINUTES TO HEALTH
SABER FUNDAMENTAL TRAINING
SAI TRAINING AND SEQUENCES
SANCHIN KATA: TRADITIONAL TRAINING FOR KARATE POWER
SCALING FORCE
SHAOLIN KUNG FU FUNDAMENTAL TRAINING: COURSES 1 & 2
SHAOLIN LONG FIST KUNG FU: ADVANCED SEQUENCES 1
SHAOLIN LONG FIST KUNG FU: ADVANCED SEQUENCES 2
SHAOLIN LONG FIST KUNG FU: BASIC SEQUENCES
SHAOLIN LONG FIST KUNG FU: INTERMEDIATE SEQUENCES
SHAOLIN SABER: BASIC SEQUENCES
SHAOLIN STAFF: BASIC SEQUENCES
SHAOLIN WHITE CRANE GONG FU BASIC TRAINING: COURSES 1 & 2
SHAOLIN WHITE CRANE GONG FU BASIC TRAINING: COURSES 3 & 4
SHUAI JIAO: KUNG FU WRESTLING
SIMPLE QIGONG EXERCISES FOR HEALTH
SIMPLE QIGONG EXERCISES FOR ARTHRITIS RELIEF
SIMPLE QIGONG EXERCISES FOR BACK PAIN RELIEF

SIMPLIFIED TAI CHI CHUAN: 24 & 48 POSTURES
SIMPLIFIED TAI CHI FOR BEGINNERS 48
SIX HEALING SOUNDS
SUN TAI CHI
SUNRISE TAI CHI
SUNSET TAI CHI
SWORD: FUNDAMENTAL TRAINING
TAEKWONDO KORYO POOMSAE
TAI CHI BALL QIGONG: COURSES 1 & 2
TAI CHI BALL QIGONG: COURSES 3 & 4
TAI CHI BALL WORKOUT FOR BEGINNERS
TAI CHI CHUAN CLASSICAL YANG STYLE
TAI CHI CONNECTIONS
TAI CHI ENERGY PATTERNS
TAI CHI FIGHTING SET
TAI CHI FIT: 24 FORM
TAI CHI FIT: FLOW
TAI CHI FIT: FUSION BAMBOO
TAI CHI FIT: FUSION FIRE
TAI CHI FIT: FUSION IRON
TAI CHI FIT: HEART HEALTH WORKOUT
TAI CHI FIT IN PARADISE
TAI CHI FIT: OVER 50
TAI CHI FIT OVER 50: BALANCE EXERCISES
TAI CHI FIT OVER 50: SEATED WORKOUT
TAI CHI FIT OVER 60: GENTLE EXERCISES
TAI CHI FIT OVER 60: HEALTHY JOINTS
TAI CHI FIT OVER 60: LIVE LONGER
TAI CHI FIT: STRENGTH
TAI CHI FIT: TO GO
TAI CHI FOR WOMEN
TAI CHI FUSION: FIRE
TAI CHI QIGONG
TAI CHI PUSHING HANDS: COURSES 1 & 2
TAI CHI PUSHING HANDS: COURSES 3 & 4
TAI CHI SWORD: CLASSICAL YANG STYLE
TAI CHI SWORD FOR BEGINNERS
TAI CHI SYMBOL: YIN YANG STICKING HANDS
TAIJI & SHAOLIN STAFF: FUNDAMENTAL TRAINING
TAIJI CHIN NA IN-DEPTH
TAIJI 37 POSTURES MARTIAL APPLICATIONS
TAIJI SABER CLASSICAL YANG STYLE
TAIJI WRESTLING
TRAINING FOR SUDDEN VIOLENCE
UNDERSTANDING QIGONG 1: WHAT IS QI? • HUMAN QI
    CIRCULATORY SYSTEM
UNDERSTANDING QIGONG 2: KEY POINTS • QIGONG BREATHING
UNDERSTANDING QIGONG 3: EMBRYONIC BREATHING
UNDERSTANDING QIGONG 4: FOUR SEASONS QIGONG
UNDERSTANDING QIGONG 5: SMALL CIRCULATION
UNDERSTANDING QIGONG 6: MARTIAL QIGONG BREATHING
WATER STYLE FOR BEGINNERS
WHITE CRANE HARD & SOFT QIGONG
YANG TAI CHI FOR BEGINNERS
YOQI QIGONG FOR A HAPPY HEART
YOQI QIGONG FOR HAPPY SPLEEN & STOMACH
YOQI QIGONG FOR HAPPY KIDNEYS
YOQI QIGONG FLOW FOR HAPPY LUNGS
YOQI QIGONG FLOW FOR STRESS RELIEF
YOQI SIX HEALING SOUNDS
WU TAI CHI FOR BEGINNERS
WUDANG KUNG FU: FUNDAMENTAL TRAINING
WUDANG SWORD
WUDANG TAIJIQUAN
XINGYIQUAN
YANG TAI CHI FOR BEGINNERS

more products available from . . .

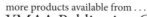

YMAA Publication Center, Inc. 楊氏東方文化出版中心

1-800-669-8892 • info@ymaa.com • www.ymaa.com